Autism
with
HEART

A Guide for Parents with Newly Diagnosed Kids

Katherine Kanaaneh

ISBN-10: 1539783650
ISBN-13: 978-1539783657

Bonus Material

Download the five free bonuses that accompany this book at: www.AutismMomMindset.com/downloads

1. Peace of Mind Checklist

2. Morning Checklist

3. Contact Log

4. Master Contact and ICE Lists

5. Insurance Reimbursement Process

To my Mom and Dad, Linda & Nathan Takeuchi, for giving me my first journal when I was 6 years old and inspiring me to write.

To my children Tim, Callia and Zara… always remember to be true to yourself, love one another, and shine.

To my husband, Ty, thank you for being strong enough for both of us at times.

To my fellow Autism Moms, celebrate the little things; it is my sincere hope that it will lead you to a greater life for you and your family

Table of Contents

Chapter 1
Introduction

*"What you do every day matters more than
what you do once in a while."*
—Gretchen Rubin

Are you overwhelmed by the demands and stress of parenting a child with autism? Are you submerged in paperwork from your school district, insurance company, and the multitude of reports related to your child's diagnosis? Moms of kids with autism lead stressful lives trying to navigate autism best practices, handle daily struggles, manage their child's therapies, contend with housework, and deal with insurance companies, school districts and so on.

Your to do list is endless, and on top of nurturing your child with autism, you may also be taking care of other children, an aging parent, or spouse; or here's a crazy thought – finding time for yourself. When was the last time you felt in control of your life and had free time to do what you wanted to do not something that you had to do?

Since this book specifically helps parents—who despite wanting to help their child, feel overwhelmed with the demands that come with parenting a special needs child—it will give you tools to manage your stress and guide you in systemizing your home so you have time for YOU.

My son was diagnosed ten years ago (at three years old) and has run the gamut of behaviors and sensory needs. His sister was less than a year old at the time, and I stayed up late at night researching online, trying to figure out ways to help my son. With this constant stress and lack of sleep, I was tired, scared, and on edge most of the time. I want to share what I've learned over the last ten years to help my family live a greater life.

Moms of special needs kids can learn to be truly present in their daily lives, have more time to themselves, and be their best self by implementing the H.E.A.R.T. Method. Since you, as a mom of a child with autism, have many demands on your plate, the steps are presented in bite size pieces and the chapters are arranged so it's easy to focus on the areas that are most important to you.

Jean, a special needs mom in San Jose says, "This book explains the H.E.A.R.T. Method in a concise and easy to read format. When I had a few minutes, I could read something and implement it that day with my family. As I went through the book, I learned strategies that lifted a lot of weight off my shoulders. I now have a system for all the paperwork that comes with having a child with autism and routines which make a big difference in the way I manage daily life in my home."

I promise that if you follow the steps in this book, you will have systems in place to simplify your life and have more time to yourself. Don't spend years trying to figure things out on your own while precious time is lost. You are the heart of your home. The H.E.A.R.T. Method will help you gain control of your life and your time so you can truly help your family.

The H.E.A.R.T. Method:

Step 1 – H: Heal by Learning

Step 2 – E: Energize

Step 3 – A: Anticipate

Step 4 – R: Routines

Step 5 – T: Thrive

The H.E.A.R.T. Method was designed to help parents as we are the heart of our families and homes. And it is through our journey as parents that we shape our families.

Chapter 2
A Note to the Reader

I know it's overwhelming right now. There were days I didn't know if I was going to make it out of the house because I kept crying.

Those first few weeks after the diagnosis I didn't want to see anyone. I was crying all the time; the slightest thing would cause me to tear up, but I didn't want my son to see me crying. Once when I was at the grocery store, a young boy was pointing to something, telling his Mom that he wanted it. His Mom responded that they would be having lunch as soon as they got home so he didn't need anything else. Their simple conversation pulled at my heart; it was such a simple interaction yet my son and I had never experienced it.

Looking back, I'm glad I let myself have that time to process those feelings as I would need the strength and perseverance for not just the next few months but for years to come.

Birthdays, which used to be a cause for celebration, suddenly felt like a milestone marker of all the things that my son wasn't doing yet. He wasn't communicating with us, he repeated the words from his favorite books over and over again, and he had no interest in toys or other children. With all these negative feelings, I knew I needed to do something. In order to let go of those feelings of grief and look toward a brighter future, my husband and I went and talked to someone who had a child with autism.

We learned about their son's challenges, the different therapies he did, and the progress that he made. We felt hopeful about the possibilities for our son.

Receiving an autism diagnosis is not a death sentence. Your life may have challenges that your friends of typical children will never face, but it doesn't mean that you and your family can't have a good life. A great life.

I refer to children without special needs as "typical" for lack of a better word. It sounded odd when I first heard it used ten years ago. However "typical peer" is part of the lingo used by professionals in this field, and I couldn't think of something more appropriate. I also tend to refer to a single child in the male form as it is easier to read the flow of the book versus scattering "he/she" and "his/her" throughout. This book was written as if I was talking to another Autism Mom. I realize and appreciate that you may be an Autism Dad, friend, grandparent, etc.

We all go on our unique journey to find our way and to help our child. You will learn a lot of acronyms (SPD, ATEC, GFCF, SDC, etc.) and have new vocabulary (sensory, vestibular, echolalia, etc.) thrown at you. You will learn about many different therapy options and places for your child to receive services.

You will find strategies to cope with behaviors, as I made it my first priority to help my son with his sensory issues which were impeding his learning, on my website www.AutismMomMindset.com. His sensory seeking tendencies made it difficult to sit still and attend to anything. He also had repetitive behaviors such as flapping pages on books and tapping things.

Here are some things to consider:

1. This is still the same child that you had before he received his diagnosis. I know this sounds simple, but it's a reminder that I needed for myself. I look back at some of the pictures of my son taken when he was first diagnosed, and I feel like I missed some of him because I was so focused on trying to "recover" him. If I could travel back in time, I would tell my younger self to really see and enjoy him for the fun kid that he was because the years will fly by.

2. Find a support group. You can usually find one through your local regional center or non-profit

that specializes in helping families with special needs. In my area, Parents Helping Parents is the non-profit organization that supports families with trainings, support groups, sibling groups, and even a library. There will be other parents there that will have a wealth of information on school districts, IEPs, therapists, resources, etc.

3. If you are not getting help from your local regional center, ask your pediatrician's office to help you locate one. Regional centers may go by another name depending on the state you live in. If your child is newly diagnosed and under three years old, a social worker will help you locate early intervention services.

4. Talk to other parents whom you meet in the waiting room. I met women that are my friends today while chatting in the OT's waiting room. We started having playdates and shared things that we learned along the way such as how to work on writing or other ways to engage our kids.

5. Listen and learn but don't judge the parent next to you. One of the greatest things that I've learned on this journey is that you don't know what another parent is going through.

6. Make time for the sibling(s). Try to find time each day, even if it's just 15 minutes, to focus on your other child(ren). It's easy to get caught up in the needs of your SNK (special needs kid—yes,

another acronym). However, your other child(ren) need you too.

7. Get help. If you have family nearby that can help you, that's great. I didn't have family around, so I found a high school student to come by and help me as a mother's helper for a few hours each week. This helped keep my sanity at this point in my life.

8. Take care of yourself. We tend to put everyone's needs before our own and carry the weight of the world on our shoulders. I need this daily reminder to get a decent amount of sleep each night and to do something that feeds my soul, or I go into "Crazy Lady" mode.

9. Take the pressure off. Keep in mind that how your child progresses is not a reflection of you as a parent. Comparing your child to how another child is progressing is sometimes tempting, but I don't recommend venturing down that rabbit hole. Focus on your child and celebrate each step of progress along the way.

10. Your spouse is processing and dealing with emotions related to your child's diagnosis. Try to keep this in mind and support one another.

Chapter 3
Autism Mom Mindset

"Success is the sum of small efforts,
repeated day in and day out."
—Robert Collier

This chapter will cover what I call the "Autism Mom Mindset." When I refer to "mindset," I'm referring to a person's attitude or disposition. My son's autism diagnosis has changed me, my parenting philosophy, and my mindset. I realized that my state of mind impacted my son (and the rest of my family) significantly.

Can you think of a morning when you were really stressed? Were you impatient with your child—maybe trying to rush him along to get ready? Did this lead to resistance or meltdowns from your child? The saying "If Mama ain't happy, ain't no one happy" rings true in our house. Therefore, I do what I can to have a positive mindset; this benefits my family as we all have a positive start to our day.

I noticed the impact my shift in mindset had on my children and me. Usually, the shift in mindset came from a small change that I had made which helped me to be more positive. Over time I made a lot of small changes in my life which added up to a significant change in my mindset as well as my overall well-being.

I have 3 children and my oldest child has moderate–severe autism. He has many challenges that he and we, as a family, face on a daily basis. We found that if we pushed too many things on him at once, he resisted, which frustrated us; however, if we tried to focus on a small change at a time, he was willing to try.

For example, when my son was four years old, it was time consuming and stressful to get him ready for school each day. I woke him up, fed him his breakfast, helped him get dressed, brushed his teeth and put his shoes on, and then he was off to school. This may sound simple, but I remember dreading waking him in the morning to start the process. (Partly because we were working on daily living and independence skills so he could learn how to do things on his own.) I put so much pressure on myself to teach him how to do each of these things in the morning. This led to resistance from him and a battle of wills each day.

After many mornings of feeling stressed and upset that he wasn't doing anything on his own, I realized that if anything was going to change in this scenario, it would need to start with me. My stress and anxiety were coming from a place of fear, fear that he would never progress, and he would always be so behind. With my old mindset, instead of helping him learn how to do things, I was really pressuring him to learn a lot of things all at once.

In order to take the pressure off both of us, I decided to work on just one thing. At first it was putting on his socks. I would help him do everything else without expecting much from him, but I made sure that we had extra time allotted for him to put his socks on by himself. I showed him how I put my socks on. While we went through many mornings of him not wanting to do it on his own, I stuck to the goal of having him put on his own socks. I focused on only that one thing, so I didn't stress about helping him with everything else.

I used to think that by helping him with his morning routine, he would never be able to do it on his own. Eventually, he put his socks on by himself without even thinking about it because he had gotten into the routine of doing it. Then we moved onto the next little thing that he needed to do which was to put on his shoes by himself. You get the idea...

This strategy of making one little change until it becomes a routine is so helpful that I have repeated it in different areas of my life. As different areas of my life improved, I became happier and more fulfilled as they shifted my mindset.

Today is a new day

Have you ever had one of those days where you wished it were over? I've had those days and felt so guilty because I know there are people out there that are struggling to have enough food to eat and basic human rights. Yet, here I was feeling sorry for myself because I had my second miscarriage and my two year old would not eat anything I put in front of him. He was screaming at me; he didn't have any communication skills; and he wouldn't stop crying.

There are many challenges that come with parenting a two or three year old. Add to this a child that has little to no communication skills, and a variety of sensory and behavioral challenges, and life can be hard. An autism mom whom I met in a speech therapist's office half-jokingly said that her child with autism is equal to three typical children. I knew exactly what she meant because my son (who was five years old at the time) was a sensory seeker and needed constant supervision. He couldn't sit and play on his own while I prepared lunch or even went to the bathroom.

Once I left him for a couple of minutes in the living room while I went to the bathroom, as he seemed occupied flipping through books, but when I got back, I couldn't find him. I found him in the hallway closet; he had climbed up the shelves and was lying in the towels and bedsheets. Thank goodness the shelf didn't collapse on him. Did I mention that he is a sensory seeker that also likes being up high?

I would get through those days by counting down how many hours I had until his bedtime. I knew that I would get a fresh new day tomorrow. My hope for you is that you take TODAY as your fresh new day: step back and survey your life and shine a light on all that you have to be grateful for.

When I was at my lowest points, I would go through everything I was grateful for: my health, my husband, my parents, brother, close friends, etc. From there, my thoughts would go to being grateful for other things. I thought of the freedom that we have, the community that I lived in, having fresh water every day, the sun shining outside. By the time I went through everything my brain threw out, I was ready to move forward.

I want to help you move forward as well. Do you want to do something to improve your life but don't know what to do? You stay up late trying to keep up with your life and always feel like you are behind. Your child has so many needs that need to be addressed—should you buy those sensory toys that your OT told you about, or should you call up the psychologist you heard could help? He keeps waking up every night and you need a plan there as well. You know things have to change but feel overwhelmed with all the areas needing change, so you don't know where to begin.

Small changes in your mindset add up to big changes over time; the shift can be so gradual that you don't even realize that you made a shift. Then when you look back, you are surprised at how far you have come. What if you purposefully made those small shifts in your life? Think of all the possibilities that lay before you. You will be able to see incredible changes with purposefully shifting your mindset.

I enjoy learning new ways to make small improvements in my life. I am definitely a work in progress, and although my life doesn't flow seamlessly every day, I have put systems into place so that I have strategies to help me make the most of each day. I hope this book inspires you to make little changes in your life, which will cumulatively have a big impact and help you to live a greater life.

"Whether you think you can,
or you think you can't—you're right."
—Henry Ford

Your circumstances today are what they are. With your mindset set on looking for the positive in your life and believing in yourself, you will find ways to accomplish things. Henry Ford said, "Whether you think you can, or you think you can't—you're right." I remind myself of this whenever my thoughts start getting negative as I have been down that road before. I know that the likelihood of having a positive outcome in a given situation is greatly reduced if I'm harboring negative thoughts.

I encourage you to look at your life through the eyes of someone living with challenging circumstances and thriving. Let me introduce you to Meg Zucker. She was born with a rare condition known as ectrodactyly, which left her with one finger on each hand and shortened forearms.

Her condition has not held her back from building an amazing life. She is a wife, mother, lawyer, speaker and philanthropist. She started Don't Hide It Flaunt It, which became a charity in 2015. She publishes a regular blog along with contributions from people all over the world writing about what makes them different. Meg flaunts her condition to encourage others to celebrate what makes them unique.

We all come into this world with different circumstances. Sometimes it takes stepping back to appreciate and rise above the challenges in our life.

I invite you to try this approach and look for the positives in your life and open your mind to the possibility of a greater life. Norman Vincent Peale said, "Change your thoughts and you change your world." In his book *The Power of Positive Thinking*, he gives many examples of people who changed their circumstances by shifting their mindset.

Initially, when you try anything new, it will take longer to figure out how to do things. After you've done it several times, you can go into auto pilot and not even think about it. For example, when you're cooking something from a new recipe, it takes time to pull out the ingredients and read each step for what you need to do. Once you've made this dish several times, you may not even need to refer to the recipe. You can pull out all the ingredients without thinking about it.

This is why I suggest making little changes at a time instead of trying to implement too many things at once. If you make one little change at a time, you won't feel burdened by the change. In fact, it will excite you to make another little change. However, if you make too many changes at once, you may feel overwhelmed and lose steam for making any changes at all.

As you go through this book, I recommend you do the following to get the most out of it:

1. Start each chapter with the intention of finding something useful that you can apply to your life. This is the most important step. You must believe that you can make a change; without your belief, you won't succeed. You can make a difference in your life TODAY. I tell my children when they go off to school each day, "Go shine!" because I want them to know that they are bright and beautiful and have it within them to do whatever they set their mind to. Now I'm telling you, my fellow Mom, "Go shine!" because I know that you've got it in you.

2. Select one change that you will make today and do it; it can be the smallest thing but making a change will give you a feeling of control over your life. Don't try to implement too many changes at

once, or you may be overwhelmed and give up altogether.

3. Celebrate that you made a step towards living a greater life. Check things off on the checklists as you go through the book if this gives you a sense of accomplishment (it does for me!). As I see more checkmarks, I feel a sense of accomplishment and motivation to keep moving forward.

4. Repeat the change that you made until it becomes a routine for you.

5. Celebrate the positive change that you have made in your life which is now effortless for you. After this, go back and find another change to make by repeating steps 1–4, and you will build momentum. You will find that by establishing routines, you have more time for yourself and don't have as many things running through your head.

Let's jump into the H.E.A.R.T. Method!

Step 1
H: Heal by Learning

*"What you do today can improve all
your tomorrows."*
—Ralph Marston

Have you ever scrolled through Facebook and thought how easy everyone else's life is? They're not juggling a child with autism—they are going places, having a grand time and life is great.

You, on the other hand, have a mountain of things on your plate—figuring out how to help your child on a daily basis with tantrums and/or sensory issues, and maybe even what to feed him. You're also trying to research everything from autism best practices to potential therapists or doctors, all the while learning how to submit insurance paperwork.

Having a child with autism is stressful, especially the first few years as there is so much to learn and wrap your head around. I often dreamed that it was the first day of college classes and I didn't know where I should be going. I saw everyone else walking to their classes, and I didn't even know what my next class was much less which building I should be heading towards. Apparently, I was so overwhelmed in my daily life that this emotion came through in my dreams.

A lot of the stress that I had was self-imposed. My heart felt like it had been dealt a heavy blow when we received our son's diagnosis. I knew I needed to heal my broken heart, and I found that the best way to do that was by learning. The more I learned about all things autism, the better I felt about being able to help my son. Learning about what I could do to help my son gave me a sense of control again, control that I'd felt was lost when we received his diagnosis.

Learning from experts about different therapies, resources, programs, etc., was empowering. Meeting and learning from other moms has been priceless. These are the things that I have learned through the years that have helped me. I have broken this down into the following chapters:

1. Learn from the Experts

2. Autism Overload—Organize Your Stuff

3. Build Your Tribe

I encourage you to check things off as you go through each chapter, so you can see your progress in each area throughout the book. Let's get started!

Chapter 4
Learn from the Experts

The saying "You don't know what you don't know," which has been attributed to Donald Rumsfeld, holds true in learning about autism services. This lesson becomes clear to parents especially when working with their school district. If you don't know what services are out there and what programs your school district provides, then you wouldn't know to go after them.

This is where doing your homework in advance can mean significant benefits to your child in terms of services and accommodations not only with your school district but with other programs as well. Seek recommendations on advocates, therapists, psychologists, or whatever professionals you are looking for.

I suggest you do the following:

1. Find an organization in your area that supports families with special needs. Check out the Center for Parent Information and Resources

(www.parentcenterhub.org/find-your-center/) to find the closest Parent Training and Information (PTI) Center or Community Parent Resource Center (CPRC). These organizations offer valuable information and support to parents of children with disabilities.

2. Attend an IEP workshop to learn your rights. IEP stands for Individualized Education Program. Every child who receives special education services must have an IEP. The IEP is a written document which is developed between you and your child's school district. This important document guides what special education supports and what services your child will receive. Learn as much as you can about the IEP process and your role in this process.

3. Join a local autism support group and connect with other parents. There are all kinds of autism organizations: Autism Society of America has chapters across the country. Go to their website and find the one closest to you. They have meet ups and events throughout the year as well as links to other autism organizations in the area that you may be interested in. Go to the events and learn what services are available by talking with other parents.

4. Get recommendations from the workshops that you attend. Talk with professionals as well as fellow parents attending the meetings.

5. Get on the wait list. Sadly, with so many kids needing services, there is a wait list for different providers. I suggest getting on several wait lists while you determine which one is your first choice. Sometimes your first choice is not available for 9 months and your second choice is available in 1 month. You will have some difficult decisions to make, but you need to create options for yourself. Call today to reserve your spot and get started on the paperwork that you need to complete. You will often find that the paperwork needs to be completed first in order to reserve your spot on the waiting list, so get the paperwork done as soon as possible.

6. If you live in a remote area and do not have access to a local autism support group, join an online support group. An online support group is helpful as you can ask a question and get feedback in real time from a broad audience.

The recommendations above will help you increase your knowledge about what you can do to help your child. You will learn how to advocate for your child, and as you look into the above resources, it will open the door to other opportunities.

Finding an organization in your area to get support and learn about different resources in your area is crucial for helping you now. Complete the intake forms to get your child on various providers' waiting lists.

Setting things into motion that can help your child will help reduce your stress as you go from feeling lost and alone to feeling informed and supported. As you start putting things into place for your child, you will notice that suddenly you have a lot of paperwork coming your way.

There will be assessment reports and recommendations from each of the various providers as well as your child's school district. The next chapter will go into the different reports that you may receive as well as how to organize them in a way that is easy for you to access them when you need them.

Chapter 5
Autism Overload—
Organize Your Stuff

You have started looking into support groups, signed up for an IEP workshop, and completed paperwork to get on some waiting lists. Let's go over how to organize your autism related paperwork.

When my son was first diagnosed, I had no idea how much paperwork was going to come my way. First there are the forms that you need to complete for every potential therapist, school, psychologist, advocate, lawyer, doctor, etc.

Then there are the reports that you will receive from the aforementioned individuals. Next there is the billing and receipts that you will receive from the different professionals. And finally the insurance documentation and reimbursement that goes along with it. In Chapter 16 "System for Insurance Paperwork," I lay out a system for managing all the paperwork related to insurance reimbursement so it doesn't overtake your life.

There is also paperwork related to your child's IEP that you will want to keep organized as well as other things that you may want to track for your child. (Things such as sensory issues, behavior, diet, skills acquired, etc.) The individuals and doctors that your child sees may want copies of the various reports that you have so that they can target similar goals to help your child progress.

Before my son was diagnosed, I worked as a CPA, which honed my organizational skills. I used these skills to streamline the incoming and outgoing paperwork related to my son.

So let's get you organized:

1. Create two file folders for all professional reports: hard copy file folder and computer soft copy folder. You will typically receive a hard copy report from the different doctors or professionals who assess your child. Keep the hard copy in a folder and ask for a soft copy if they don't provide you with one.

2. You will want that copy because you will need to share the different reports between your child's different providers. All the providers will want the initial diagnosis report from your child's developmental pediatrician or psychologist. Your insurance company will also need that report

from you if you are looking for insurance reimbursement for services.

3. Keep all soft copies of reports that you receive from professionals in a specific folder so you know where to find them. When you save a soft copy of the report, give it a filename that is specific to that report, and it will group together similar reports. For example, Dr. Insert Name Initial Assessment August 2016. This way if you have future reports from Dr. Insert Name and you give it a similar filename, it will group them together, and you can see the report name and the date for the report you are looking for.

   You will want to easily access these reports because even if you have a set list of providers for your child, things may change, and you will have to start this process again. Your speech therapist may no longer be an in-network provider; thus, you may want to switch over to someone who is in network for you, and now the new provider will need the reports. Be sure to back up your files to the cloud or external drive.

4. Create an IEP binder with copies of all relevant reports that you've given your school district. You will want a large sturdy binder as this binder will be holding a lot of reports. Create tabs that are relevant such as: Contact Log, Current IEP, Initial Assessment Report by SD (School District), Initial Assessment Report by Physician, SLP

Report, OT Report, etc. I kept the individual reports in plastic sleeve covers so I wouldn't have to keep unlocking and locking the binder. It was easier to access this way, and the plastic sleeve made it easy to remember which reports were removed because the empty sleeve was there as a reminder.

5. Create a Master Schedule for your family which includes all ongoing times for school, therapies, practices, tutoring, etc. This schedule should also list any relevant carpooling information. If you work full time and there is a nanny who cares for your child, your nanny will need to know where your child needs to be or whom to expect at your home for any home therapy sessions. Or if you are ill and can barely get out of bed, you will not want to explain your child's schedule to someone at that time. If it is readily available, you can just point them to the spot where you keep the info, and they can let you rest.

6. Create a Master Contact & In Case of Emergency list; you can download a free template at www.AutismMomMindset.com. This list is useful for anyone other than you who needs the contact info for your child's providers. The caregiver needs this info so they will have the contact info for whom to call in case a therapist doesn't show up. It will also list the in case of emergency information for your family, so in the event that your child has a medical emergency, your

caregiver will have your address, closest major cross street, etc. on hand if they need to call 911.

7. Keep a Contact Log of all the reports that you've submitted to your school district along with the date that you gave it to them. You can download a free template at www.AutismMomMindset.com. Store this log in your IEP binder.

I also kept a photo of my son on the front of the IEP binder which was visible to the IEP team so they could keep in mind that we are discussing my child. Advocating for your child can be challenging; therefore, having a photo of your child in front of you during IEP meetings may give you the strength you need during those times.

You now have a system for your child's autism related reports. Once you've completed this, you'll feel a sense of accomplishment for having your reports organized and at your fingertips. Pat yourself on the back for a job well done. Now let's go over a crucial area of importance for autism moms.

Chapter 6
Build Your Tribe

Your reports have been neatly filed away and are easy for you to retrieve. With one less worry on your mind, let's discuss the importance of building your tribe.

Is there a minute in the day that you aren't thinking about autism on some level? The first few years after my son was diagnosed, I lived and breathed autism. It was the first thing that I thought of each day and the last thing I thought about when I fell asleep. It was as if there were a constant, daily buzzer going off in my head, questioning whether I had done enough for my son or if I had missed something.

One of the best things that you can do to ease your stress level is to meet other moms that can relate to the challenges that you're having and share the fears that you have for your child's future. Drop in on a parent coffee for parents of children with autism or a support group meeting. These meetings are informal and a great way to connect with other parents.

If you are shy by nature and are hesitant about going to a group meeting, reach out to the support group leader. Most meetings follow one of two formats: a speaker discussing a topic relevant to the parents (topics could range from strategies to dealing with sensory issues to how to teach your child social skills or a host of other topics); or an informal format where parents just talk and connect with each other. At the informal meetings, depending on the size of the group, the support group leader will say a little something about her journey with autism and answer any questions that were brought forth from the previous meeting.

If it's a small group, the support group leader will have everyone go around the room and give her reason for being there (i.e. my name is Kat, I have a 13 year old son with autism, and I live in San Jose). Some parents may want to share what city they live in so that parents can connect with people that are near them to meet for playdates or coffee.

If you don't connect with anyone on the first meeting, I encourage you to go to a few more. People don't go to every meeting due to commitments or issues with their child so you will see some familiar faces at the next meeting and you will also meet new people. Plus, you will learn something new at each meeting; the information may not be something you need right now, but it may be something you can look into down the road if and when it applies to your child.

Do you have questions related to your child's behavior? IEP questions? Looking for ideas on how to engage your child? Looking for lawyer or advocate recommendations? Wondering if other parents take their child to restaurants? Wondering what sort of toys other kids like to play with? Whatever questions you have, bring them to the group; that's what these groups are there for: to help you, as a parent, not feel so alone.

Before you go to the meeting, grab a notebook and start jotting down questions that come to mind. If you use Evernote or another note taking app on your phone, keep a file for autism meeting questions. Any time that a question comes to mind, write it down or put it in your app, so that when you attend the meeting, you will be able to get all your questions answered.

The meeting facilitator and other parents may not have an answer to a specific question that you're looking for, but they may be able to direct you some place or to someone that can help you. I have met autism moms who have introduced me to another parent that could help me, and I've been on the other side of that as well. A friend of mine will refer another mom who has questions that she knows I can help with.

Support group meetings are usually held on a monthly basis and by volunteer parents that are also parents of children with autism. Bring that notebook or pull up that app that you are storing your questions in. Don't worry about asking too many questions, your questions will help not only you but the person sitting next to you.

If nothing else, going to a monthly support group meeting allows you time to take a break from being a caregiver for a couple of hours. The meeting allows you to surround yourself with other parents that are navigating this new world just like you.

Eventually, you may not feel the need to attend group meetings anymore, but hopefully you have met another mom or two that you connected with and that you consider part of your tribe. Trust me, when the going gets tough with the ups and downs of life with autism, a friend that shares a similar journey can offer insight that no one else can.

Your tribe will be there to share different things along the way such as how they handle challenging behaviors or what they are doing to prepare their child for going on an airplane. You may be potty training at the same time or all learning to manage the challenges that come with puberty.

Just listening to one of my fellow autism moms talk about something that her child is going through normalizes my own life for me, reminding me I am not alone in this journey. And neither are you.

I am not recommending that you shun your friends that don't have a child with autism; I'm recommending that you find at least one person that shares a similar journey. Having a friend that you can bounce ideas off or share resources with will help you to feel less isolated.

Having a tribe is fundamentally important for healing your heart, easing your stress level, and learning new ways for you to help your child. Let's move on to the next step of the H.E.A.R.T. method—E for Energize.

Step 2
E: Energize

*"To discern what is truly essential
we need space to think, time to look and
listen, permission to play, wisdom to sleep,
and the discipline to apply highly selective
criteria to the choices we make."*
—Greg McKeown

In the first step, we covered different ways to heal by learning. Hopefully, you are regaining a sense of control in your life as you learn different ways to help your child. Your autism-related reports all have a home now, and you can easily access them in soft and hard copy. You have started building your tribe which will help with the stress that comes with a diagnosis. Now it's time to go over what you can do to clarify what is important in your life. By doing this, you will be able to get some time back in your day for other things. Who doesn't want that?

This step will cover key things that you can do in your life to energize yourself so that you can make the most out of each day. Before I proceed, I would like to remember the advice given in the earlier chapter on mindset (Chapter 3): start each chapter with the intention of finding something useful that you can apply to your life.

I wish that I had incorporated these practices into my life a long time ago, but I felt they would be a drain on me. I didn't understand how adding something to my life could make the other things in my life so much simpler. After consistently incorporating these practices into my life, I have found them to be uplifting and beneficial for helping me to clarify what is truly important for my family and me.

Energize Framework:

1. Recharge Your Batteries

2. Get off the Phone (Or Email in this Case!)

3. Give Thanks

4. Find Peace

Give each of these changes and enriching practices a good two week trial (at a minimum), and see if they make a difference in your life. Let's get started.

Chapter 7
Recharge Your Batteries

We've gone over a lot of things for you to learn in a short amount of time—what and how to learn from the experts and other parents as well as how to organize your autism related paperwork. In the beginning, you are quickly trying to learn and get your child squared away with the proper therapies, getting a handle on all the paperwork, managing your child's new schedule, and emotionally wrapping your head around all the changes going on around you.

Now I'm going to tell you to do something which sounds completely counter intuitive, but I want you to hear me out. Deal? Okay… I want you to go to bed early tonight. "What?" you ask, how can I go to bed early when I have a gazillion things on my plate to figure out. Let me explain by example.

When my son was starting different therapies as well as a new school, I was also caring for his toddler sister, and on top of all that, I was fighting insurance claims, dealing with feeding challenges with my son, and so on. Dealing with one of those things and the demands of daily life is manageable. However, enduring all of those challenges at once, budgeting lots of new expenses, and giving up my job to manage my son's new program took me to the tipping point. Sometimes my heart would be pounding so hard in my chest that I was sure I was on the verge of a health crisis.

It was at these stressful times that I wanted to clear clutter. Suddenly, nothing was more important to me than clearing the stack of papers that had piled up on my dining room table. Other times, it would be my main desk drawer or the top of my desk—I had to clean it up, or I couldn't do anything else.

Looking back, I can see that I avoided the things that needed my attention because I felt overwhelmed and just wanted it to go away on its own. Instead, I focused on something easier that was within my control but wasn't a priority at that moment.

My to do list didn't go away on its own but delaying doing what needed to be done caused me to stay up late. I would stay up researching on my computer even though I should have been going to bed. I would be at the computer searching for the answer for "one more thing" and would even be falling asleep in the process.

This meant that I was tired AND grouchy the next day. I was not my best self, and I realized that if I kept doing what I was doing, I would be letting my children and myself down. I wasn't giving them my best self every day, just a fraction of my scattered self.

It was during this time in my life that I began figuring out a system to manage the overwhelming paperwork. Everything piling on my plate on top of this paperwork felt like too much.

With so much to do, I know how hard it is to go to bed at a decent hour; I have always been a night owl and stayed up late. Yet, I paid a high price for my chronic lack of sleep as I was not my best self during the day and could quickly spiral down into Crazy Lady Mode (more on that in Chapter 13 If All Else Fails). I found myself losing my temper often and not liking the Mom that I had become. I wanted my kids to have a Mom that was fun, loving, and patient with them. I needed to stop sleepwalking through the day and really show up as the mom that my kids deserved.

Many studies and books have shown how important sleep is for our learning, immune function, and other vital areas in our lives. Lack of sleep may affect our health, safety, and even our longevity. Needless to say, sleep is crucial for having the energy you need each day. In order to get a good night's sleep, it is important you make it a priority.

When you miss a good night's rest here or there, you can function during the day. However, when you repeat this cycle over and over, the lack of sleep catches up with you. Most parents prioritize sleep for their children as they have seen their children's behavior when they haven't been getting a good night's rest. As parents, we focus on our children's sleep by having a set bedtime and sleep ritual for them. We put on their pajamas, brush their teeth, read bedtime stories, give goodnight kisses, and ease them into bed.

Parents should prioritize their own sleep schedule by doing the same things for themselves. Set your bedtime and sleep ritual so that you will have a good night's rest as well. If you are a night owl like I was, I suggest setting your bedtime for 30 minutes before you usually go to bed. You may want to set a timer to remind you every night to start your sleep ritual. This is easy to do with a smartphone; you can set your alarm to go off every night to let you know that it's time to get ready for bed.

You may intend to go to bed at a certain time, but you can get distracted by whatever you are doing. By having that alarm go off every night, it reminds you that you have prioritized sleep and should start getting ready for bed. Without that nightly alarm, you may lose track of the time and stay up later.

Here are a few suggestions for creating a sleep ritual if getting to bed is difficult for you:

1. It's difficult to fall asleep when you are worrying about what you have to do the next day. Make sure you have done your night time prep (we will cover this in chapter 14 Peace of Mind Routine) before you start your sleep ritual so that you are prepared for tomorrow.

2. Prepare for bed when you're getting your kids ready for bed or shortly thereafter. If you need to take out your contacts, wash your face, and brush your teeth before bed, do these things when your kids are getting ready for bed. If you can't do it when your kids are getting ready for bed because they need your help, then do these things as soon as you've put them to sleep. This will make it easier for you to go to bed when it's your bedtime as you will have already gotten many of the bedtime steps out of the way.

3. Cool down your bedroom; you may want to sleep with a fan on. The sound of the fan is also good white noise to aid in helping you fall asleep. Set the temperature of your thermostat to drop down to your desired temperature before you get to bed so the room is already nice and cool when you are ready to go to sleep. The temperature of your sleep area will affect the quality of your sleep because your body temperature goes down when you sleep. However, finding the right temperature varies from person to person. The typical range is between 65 and 72 degrees Fahrenheit.

4. Dim the lights as you're getting ready for bed. If your room is fully lit as you're getting ready for bed, it takes a while for you to adjust to a dark room. However, if the lights are dimmed as you're getting ready for bed, it's an easier transition into sleep mode.

5. Darken the room by using block out shades or films if your room let's in the light from outside. If this is difficult, you can sleep with an eye cover to block out the light.

I hope you go to bed early and give yourself the gift of waking up refreshed and ready to meet the day. Sometimes when you're so tired every day, you forget what it feels like to be fully refreshed and thinking clearly during the day.

As you start going to bed at a regular time and getting more sleep each night, you will find that you have more patience with your child and can make decisions quicker. This leads to not only getting more things done that you need to get done during the day, but it also leads to a greater sense of satisfaction when you go to sleep at night knowing that you had a meaningful day.

As I said in the beginning of this chapter, I know this advice sounds counter intuitive—go to bed early even though you have so many things needing your attention. In Chapter 14 Peace of Mind Routine, I will show you routines and systems which will help things flow better during your day so you will be able to go to bed earlier without feeling like you left so many things undone.

Trust me, if you go to bed on time and wake up refreshed, you won't think to yourself, "Gee I wish I had stayed up later!" Think about how many times you have woken up tired and barely functioning, were you glad that you stayed up late the night before?

For now, trust me when I tell you that going to bed earlier is something that I rarely did, and I paid the price. My husband used to tell me I needed to get to bed because I would pay for it the next day, and he was right. It has taken me years to learn this lesson. I hope that you will incorporate this change into your life and reap the many benefits from getting a good night's sleep.

Now, I want to introduce you to something that will save you time every day. More importantly, it will save you from mentally thinking about it throughout your day and give you the freedom to focus on more important things.

Chapter 8
Get Off the Phone
(Or Email in This Case!)

How much time do you spend on your email each day? My email was at 6,457 emails in my inbox AFTER I had taken about an hour and a half to clean it up. Yes, this is the result of cleaning up: I still had 6,457 emails sitting in my inbox. Never mind the other hundreds of emails that I had sitting in various folders.

Then I signed up for my free trial of Sanebox, thanks to a podcast. Sanebox isn't free, but they do offer a free 14 day trial. I figured I had nothing to lose so I signed up that night. The next morning when I went to check my email, I had fewer than 2,700 emails in my inbox. Whoa—amazing!

I reviewed what Sanebox had moved to the other folders and was impressed. Sanebox uses algorithms to determine where your emails should go and only keeps the most relevant ones in your inbox. The other emails get moved to a separate folder called SaneLater. The emails that I get from businesses go there as well as newsletters from different organizations.

You can train any email to go to the SaneLater folder. Let's say your Great Aunt Becky forwards you email every day that has jokes in it. You don't want Great Aunt Becky's emails cluttering your inbox. All you have to do is train one email from Great Aunt Becky to go to the SaneLater folder. All future emails from Great Aunt Becky will go to the SaneLater folder—it's that simple.

Two days later, after sorting through my inbox, I was able to get my inbox down to a manageable 20 emails. If you're getting email from a business or person that you don't want to see, you can train Sanebox to never allow it into your inbox again. How do you do this? By moving an email to a folder called SaneBlackhole. Once you put an email into the SaneBlackhole folder, you never have to see email coming from that person/company again. How awesome is that? Love it!

Sanebox works amazingly well and has saved me a lot of time. I don't have to go scrolling up and down through my email looking for important messages. Now I don't even need to go into my email to see if there are important emails because I don't have hundreds of unread emails in my inbox anymore. Prior to using Sanebox, the number of unread emails didn't mean anything to me because it was so high that I never knew what it was. I have spent at least eight hours on two

Christmas vacations clearing out email. Now I can't imagine wasting my vacation time going through email.

I now keep my unread emails in my inbox at zero so I know that any unread email has some significance. Thus, I no longer have to check my email whenever I have a spare moment. I can focus on what I want to focus on instead.

Sanebox is like having a personal assistant setting the important things for your review and not bothering you with non-priority items.

If I had to guess, Sanebox has saved me close to an hour a day, and I think that's a conservative estimate. That adds up to 365 hours a year because hey, I check my email every day, do you? This breaks down to 15 days a year of my time thanks to Sanebox. I feel like I am an infomercial for their company, but I am blown away by the results of this simple change.

In fact, I started writing this book about two weeks before I started using Sanebox. On day 3 of using Sanebox, I have written more than I did the two weeks before combined. I now have the time and energy that I was wasting in my email to use for something that matters to me.

Along with freeing up some time, I no longer feel weighted down by checking all those emails. It is out of my head, and it feels like a huge burden has lifted from my shoulders.

Here's what you can do:

1. Ask yourself if you're willing to commit 14 days to reduce your email once and for all. If the answer is yes, proceed to the next step.

2. Sign up for the free 14 day trial of Sanebox by going to www.sanebox.com/AutismMom and get $5 off if you decide to sign up for Sanebox once your trial period is over. Please note that this is a referral code.

3. Yay, you're signed up! Sanebox has cleaned up your inbox and created new folders for you. Now you should review the folders to ensure that nothing important to you went into the SaneLater folder. If anything important went to the SaneLater folder, then now is the time to move it to your inbox. This is how you train Sanebox to sort which emails belong in your inbox and which ones can be put into the SaneLater folder.

4. Clear out your inbox. I'm sure there are still several items in your inbox that haven't been moved to the SaneLater folder but should be moved there. Remind yourself that this little bit of time investment now will pay off once you've reduced your inbox.

5. Your inbox should now be at ZERO, and you can spend less time in your email each day. You no longer have your inbox lurking in the back of your mind because it is clean!

If you don't LOVE Sanebox by the end of your 14 day trial period, then don't sign up for their plan. They don't have your credit card information so you don't have to worry about them charging you.

Hopefully, you love Sanebox as much as I do and have more time and energy each day that you were spending on email. Let's put some of that time to use in order to shift your focus from a survival mindset to a thriving mindset.

Chapter 9
Give Thanks

My Grandma used to say, "I'm very lucky, my family is healthy and no one is in jail." I used to smile when she said that, but you know something, I think my Grandma was right.

Studies have shown that gratitude is associated with greater happiness. Dr. Robert A. Emmons of the University of California, Davis, a leading scientific expert on gratitude, explains how important gratitude is when someone is in dire circumstances. "My response is that not only will a grateful attitude help—it is essential. In fact, it is precisely under crisis conditions when we have the most to gain by a grateful perspective on life. In the face of demoralization, gratitude has the power to energize. In the face of brokenness, gratitude has the power to heal. In the face of despair, gratitude has the power to bring hope. In other words, gratitude can help us cope with hard times."

Now if that isn't a strong argument for parents with newly diagnosed kids to start practicing gratitude, I don't know what is. I tried starting a gratitude practice about 6 years ago, but it never stuck because I never found a set time to devote to it.

If you plan to do something whenever you "find the time," chances are you will never "find the time."

Including a moment to practice gratitude as part of your Morning Routine or Peace of Mind Routine (covered in Step 4 on Routines) will increase the likelihood of following through with it. If a daily commitment is too much, you could commit to every Saturday or Sunday morning when you first wake up or whatever time works for you. It doesn't matter when you pick to do it, but pick a time and stick to it.

Here's what you can do to get started:

1. Select a notebook for your gratitude journal. This doesn't have to be anything fancy. My first gratitude journal was an old notebook that I had from years ago but never used. If you prefer to use an app, I enjoy using 5 Minute Journal.

    5 Minute Journal gives you an inspiring quote each day and asks what you're grateful for and

how you could have made the day even better. I like this second question because it causes you to pause and think how you could have made the day better. And it may plant the seed in your head for a positive change you can make the next day.

2. Pick a specific time (i.e. first thing when you wake up or when you are drinking your first cup of coffee) for when you will record what you are grateful for, and that way every day when you get your first cup of coffee or tea, you will instinctively jot down something that you're grateful for.

3. In your gratitude journal or app, jot down the date (you won't need to do this in the app) and one thing that you are grateful for TODAY. Do this every day for a week; don't worry about doing more than that. You just want to get into the routine of doing it.

4. Do the same thing as above, except write down the date and two things that you are grateful for today. Do this every day for a week.

5. Do the same thing as above, except write down the date and three things that you are grateful for today. Do this every day for a week.

6. Write down the date and three things that you are grateful for today, and then read a previous gratitude journal entry. Ideally, you will have 3 weeks of journal entries. Go back to the very first

one and read it. Tomorrow after you write down your 3 things you are grateful for, read your journal entry from day two of your gratitude journal.

Once you have established this routine as a daily practice, you will find that it helps you shape your mindset to a positive one throughout the day. Your mind unconsciously starts looking for the good, even seeking it out, in your life. This is how a gratitude practice helps to energize you; it replaces those negative draining thoughts in your head with positive ones.

At this point, you have made a lot of changes in your life. You should be getting into a rhythm with these little changes incorporated into your daily routine. They should be such a part of your daily routine, such as waking up and brushing your teeth, that you don't even think about them because you naturally do them every day.

Chapter 10
Find Peace

When your child is first diagnosed, you feel overwhelmed as the diagnosis takes over your thoughts. Taking a moment each day to shift your thoughts to things that you're grateful for helps train your mind to look for the good in your life. By doing this, you stay grounded rather than swept away by stress.

Meditation is another practice you can do which reduces stress, leads to greater focus and creativity, and a host of other benefits. Hold on, don't skip this section! I know what you're thinking… 'meditation is for people that think they're such deep thinkers or oh so spiritual.' Right? Or maybe I'm the only person that had that thought flit through her head? Please stick with me on this one because meditation is one of those things that can help you have those zen moments that can seem so out of reach.

My son's behaviors are unpredictable: he could be in an upswing and doing well, appearing happy and at ease; then he does something for seemingly no reason, and I'm at a loss for what caused him to do what he did. The stress that comes with constantly monitoring someone can take its toll on you—mentally and physically.

I have found that doing a short meditation each morning instills a feeling of being "grounded" when I do it and somewhat unsettled if I don't. By grounded, I mean that I feel more in tune with myself, settled, and in control of my emotions. I can handle situations in a positive way rather than flying off the handle at the smallest thing. It is worth the effort of taking five minutes to do it because those five minutes of sitting in stillness eases me into a calmer day altogether.

Have you found a quiet place and tried it? Or did you try it while you were multi-tasking and doing something else—say, putting your child down for a nap, but you can still hear him in the background? Did you try several times over the years, but you could never stick with it? Do you think this is something you should be doing but feel so stretched you don't have time to sit still?

Looking back, I realize I held back from taking up a meditation practice (sounds so serious, huh?) mostly because I didn't know what sort of meditation to do. I also didn't have the time to look for one, and I thought it would take at least 10 minutes of my day to do the meditation. And then inspiration struck! I got the Meditation app by Gaiam free from Starbucks.

Starbucks often has free apps that they give away at the counter or through their Starbucks app. The Gaiam app has a course on "meditation essentials" which are listening bites (roughly 5–10 minutes each), so I could finally learn how to do this "meditation thing" rather than feel like I'm trying to do something but really I'm clueless.

I went through the course, and then went through what they call their "collections" of meditations. The collections are broken down into different categories for stress, sleep, anxiety, happiness, confidence, compassion, etc. Each category has short meditations in them with the length of time listed next to them. This makes it easy to pick a meditation based on how you're feeling and how much time you have.

They also have a category for "quick breaks" which is great for when you only have 2–3 minutes. Within quick breaks you can choose from timely meditations such as anger break, soften and relax, easing stress, unexpected grief, etc.

Here's what you do:

1. Download a meditation app. I recommend Gaiam or Omvana; you can find them in the app store on iTunes.

2. Pick a specific time, such as first thing when you wake up or right after you brush your teeth, for when you will do your meditation.

3. Listen to the "Starting Your Practice" lesson in the Meditation Essentials course. Continue each day and listen to one course a day; they are short lessons that provide insight into creating a meditation practice. Once you've completed the Meditation Essentials course, you should start feeling the benefits of setting aside time each day for stillness. If for some reason, this course is no longer available, try another beginner's meditation.

4. Go into the collections that are in the app, take a look at the different categories such as stress, sleep, anxiety, pain, confidence, compassion. Try out the ones that interest you.

5. Find your personal collection of favorite meditations that you can use each day to help you live a greater life.

Now you have a plan in place to energize yourself on a daily basis. You also have the tools to find more time in your day by minimizing the amount of time spent on email. Let's move on to how you can gain even more time in your day by anticipating and planning for your day to day life rather than reacting to it.

Step 3
A: Anticipate

"You build on failure. You use it as a stepping stone. Close the door on the past. You don't try to forget the mistakes, but you don't dwell on it. You don't let it have any of your energy, or any of your time, or any of your space. If you analyze it as you're moving forward, you'll never fall in the same trap twice."
—Johnny Cash

Our son was an active little boy who had a fleeting attention span. He was a sensory seeker and had a fascination with water. These qualities made things difficult when I was nursing his younger sister or trying to put her down to bed. Even going to the bathroom could spell disaster because I didn't know what awaited me when I returned. He may have taken the caps off the soap dispenser, dishwashing liquid, or even my moisturizer, and dumped them out.

It's exhausting having to clean up after your child each day. Moreover, it's frustrating knowing that you're in a vicious cycle of constant monitoring: disaster averted—relief; disaster found—oh no, clean up the mess; repeat. I unfortunately knew this song and dance far too well and knew I needed to figure out a way to break the cycle or at least minimize it.

This step is all about anticipating what typically happens during the day in your daily song and dance and putting things in place to switch things up.

Chapter 11
Zen Zone = Happy Home

Are you enjoying the freedom that Sanebox has given you? I am grateful every day for this wonderful email system; it has changed my life more than I imagined it would. Let's put some of that time that was previously spent on email to good use. This little bit of time investment now will free up more time for you going forward.

"Outer order contributes to inner calm"
—Gretchen Rubin

"Outer order contributes to inner calm" is one of author Gretchen Rubin's "secrets of adulthood." I couldn't agree more with this statement. When I look around my home and see a big mess, I feel mentally disorganized. There is a constant sense of overwhelm when I see things scattered all over my house. There could be a jacket on the counter, shoes in the entryway, a pair of socks by the stairway, a doll and some books right in the middle of the family room.

This sense of mental disorganization and overwhelm is not limited to just you, your child feels it too. In this chapter, I will give you tips on how to clear the clutter from your home to anticipate your child's needs and behaviors. You may be surprised at how much this clutter affects your state of mind once you clear it out of your home.

Sometimes it's hard to see clutter in our own homes because we see it every day. Imagine walking into an office for a job interview. The first office that you walk into you almost trip on a delivery box that is sitting in the entryway. The waiting room is strewn with magazines by previous visitors. As you walk through the office, you see a copy machine with empty boxes around it, further along the corridor you see recycle bins that are overflowing.

The next company that you go to interview with has a tidy waiting area with a few magazines neatly stacked on a table. As you walk through the office, you see that the hallways are clear and everything flows well in this space.

This example may seem a bit exaggerated, but you get the idea. Now I want you to go through an exercise: go to your front door and step outside and close the door behind you. Now with fresh eyes, as if you are a guest entering your home for the first time, step through and see your house for the first time. What do you see?

Are there things in the entryway or in the living room that are scattered about? How about the kitchen—is everything in its place or are there things everywhere? Is the kitchen table a clean inviting space to share a meal? Is it a place for your child to do an activity or is it covered with papers and other items?

For my family, we need to keep a reign on our things because my son's behaviors can be erratic at times. The more things we have out, the more potential things that he may get into. For example, one of his go to behaviors is to dump drinks. He is usually okay if we are sitting down and eating together. However, if you leave your cup on the kitchen counter and walk away, don't expect that it will be where you left it when you get back. In our house, we affectionately call that a "rookie" mistake.

Having more stuff out, especially in the main living areas, meant that there was more stuff to clean up and also more stuff that my son may get into. My middle daughter loved to draw in different notebooks when she was younger and she shared an art table with her brother that had coloring books on it. My son didn't distinguish between the coloring book and her notebook, so he colored all over it. She learned at a young age to put her special things away in her room.

Baby proofing your home for a toddler is important. It takes even more thought when you are child proofing your home for a four or five year old that can climb and has the dexterity to get into things. We put all our cleaning supplies into big baby proof containers which have a difficult latch in the front to open it.

Our old house was a ranch style home. To keep our son in the main living area when he was younger, we installed hook latches on the outside of the doors so that we could prevent him from going into the bedrooms. Without these latches, if I went to the bathroom even for a minute, I wasn't sure what I would find when I got back.

Clutter makes a big difference for my state of mind. I enjoyed reading two books on the subject: *The Life-changing Magic of Tidying Up* by Marie Kondo and *It's Here... Somewhere* by Alice Fulton-Osborne and Pauline Hatch. These books helped me look at my home with a fresh set of eyes. Let me share with you the process I use based on what I learned from those books.

1. Grab two bags and a clothes basket. Write "trash" on one bag and "donate" on the second bag. The clothes basket will hold the two bags as well as anything that doesn't belong in the room that you are clearing. Set your timer for 15 minutes and start with the room that you spend the most time in. Grab what is out in the open that applies to each of these bags and basket. You are doing this first to build excitement for this task as well as satisfaction for clearing out 2 bags of stuff in a

short amount of time. This task is best done alone without anyone questioning what you are putting in the different bags and slowing you down.

When you're done, throw the garbage away and put the donation bag somewhere that other family members won't inadvertently take things and sneak them back into the house. I usually keep the donation bags in the garage, but I found that my middle daughter was sneaking things back into the house. Before you put away the basket, take note of what is in it. You may find that designating a place for these things will help lessen future clean ups.

For example, at our old house, we had a large hanging coat rack in our laundry room to hang our coats. Our new house didn't have a good spot to hang our jackets and the closest coat closet wasn't near the door so jackets ended up in the entryway. To solve this problem, I bought a large basket that we toss our jackets into when we get home.

2. The next day you will repeat the same things that you did in #1 above. This may not take you the full 15 minutes since you cleared out the visible items yesterday. Therefore, you should use your leftover time to clear the room that your child spends the most time in. This area should be prioritized in order for your child to feel a sense of calm in his preferred space. This may be your

child's bedroom or living room, if he started a home therapy program and you're using these rooms to do most of his therapy.

3. The next day you will repeat the same thing that you did in #1 but use the entire time in the area/room that your child spends the most time in. Set your timer for 30 minutes. If everything is visibly clear, then start on the dresser. Take everything out of the dresser and before putting it back into the dresser, sort everything—short sleeved shirts together, shorts together, underwear, etc.

Anything that has a hole in it, doesn't fit, doesn't have the matching pair, or you just plain don't like toss it into one of the bags. If you find that you have way too much of something, decide how many you really need.

If you have ten t-shirts that fit and are in good shape but really only need five shirts, then toss the other five into the donate bag. This is where I find Marie Kondo's advice incredibly helpful. She suggests that you pick up each item one at a time and ask yourself if it "sparks joy" in you. It is amazing how much clarity you feel towards your "stuff" when you go through this exercise.

Your child should have much less t-shirts, jeans, etc. after you have gone through this exercise. Now fold everything and put them away, keeping like items together. Stand back and admire how great the dresser looks now. It's not overflowing, and you can see all your things without the extras (that you never used anyway) in there. You are a rock star—doesn't it feel good to clear out stuff that you weren't using?

4. The next day you will repeat the process that you did in #3 above and clean out anything else that needs to be cleaned out in this room such as the closet. If this seems like a daunting task, break it apart. Set your timer for 30 minutes and repeat this process for a section of the closet, such as the items that are on the floor of the closet or the clothes that are hanging.

If you come across something that is broken, ask yourself if you will ever have the time to fix it. Also think about the cost of fixing it vs buying a new one; even if you fix something that's broken, it may not have all the features of the new version of that item.

When you first start clearing out your stuff, you may come across items that you are unsure about; this is normal. Letting go of our stuff is hard because it is not just the physical item that we're letting go of, but the emotions we've attached to it. If you need a visual reminder to remember something, then take some pictures of the item or a picture of you or your child holding it. This may help you let go of things.

If you find something that you would like to keep as an heirloom, put it in a designated area. I keep an heirloom box for each of my kids; it is just a plastic bin that I keep their special items in.

Often the reason why it's hard to get rid of things is because we feel that we paid our hard earned money for something, and it would be a "waste" to get rid of it. Yet the price of holding onto things that we don't need only serves to clutter our lives taking not only physical space but mental space.

Can you think of a time when you were putting your clothes away and the drawers were over flowing? You saw some things that didn't really fit you anymore but you once loved. You saw something else that you bought on sale and have never worn but maybe you would wear it one day.

I encourage you to take items out that don't fit you and items you got at a great price yet you've never worn. These items are taking up physical space in your closet and mental space every time you look at them when you're trying to find what you want to wear each day. The clothes that fit you well and make you feel good should be what you have left in your closet.

When you're done, you should look back on the last four days and celebrate. You have cleaned out four bags of garbage and have four bags of stuff for donation. You also have de-cluttered an area and made it easier for you to clean and put things away because it's not overflowing with extra stuff. You are awesome!

5. Go through your home room by room and repeat the process above. Here are a few things to keep in mind. If you have certain things that are kept in different places in the house, consider consolidating them into one spot if that makes sense for your family. For instance, we had books all over our home.

We went through the books one by one and threw away the ones that were falling apart (some of our kids' books were over 10 years old and well loved) and donated the ones that we were not going to read again. Then we separated them by putting the adult books and older chapter books in one room, and the kids' early reader and picture books in the family room where the kids usually are. This makes it easier to find the book that you're looking for and also makes clean up time easier.

As I was deciding what to do with a particular item, it helped to keep in mind that someone out there could use this item. This was usually enough for me to donate something; I didn't need to hold onto it especially knowing that someone else could use it.

6. Set your calendar every quarter to go through this process room by room. It gets easier the more you do it because you realize all the benefits of having less stuff (that weren't being used) lying around the house. You also don't miss the things that you let go of; instead, it's like a weight lifted off your shoulders every time the bags of garbage and donations leave your home.

7. Train your family to put things away as soon as they are done with something. I will cover this further in Chapter 17 Life Skills & Chores. As soon as my kids walk into the house, they know that they should put their shoes into the shoe cabinet so it's not scattered in our entryway. Ironically, the biggest offender is my husband, hmm...

8. Finally, the last and most important step in this whole process is to think through what you are thinking of buying next. Do you love this item that you are thinking of purchasing? Are you sure that you don't already have something like it? Do you know where you're going to put it if you buy it?

You now have an easy to follow process to significantly reduce the amount of clutter in your home. But wait, I haven't even mentioned what to do with the paper piles. The mail, the insurance paperwork, and the reports—this can lead to piles of paper everywhere.

In Chapter 16 System for Insurance Paperwork, I will show you a system for handling the paper overload—what to do with all the reports, forms, insurance billing and more. For now, breathe because you have cleared out the clutter and made room for a greater life. In the next chapter, you will learn how to clear the mental clutter out of your head.

Chapter 12
Free Your Mind, Free Your Time

Now that you've got a system to clear the physical clutter in your home, let's put a system into place to clear out the mental clutter. What do I mean by mental clutter? Mental clutter is the thoughts that are constantly running through your head that prevent you from focusing on what is most important in your life.

Your mind is continuously thinking about all the things that you need to do each day. You often think things like, 'I need to call the therapist to see where my child is on the waitlist; what can I do to help my child with this new behavior; should I run to Home Depot to fix something in my house or should I hire a handyman; what's for dinner tonight; what else do I need from the grocery store', etc. These thoughts in our heads keep us from focusing on what we want to focus on. It's hard to be present with those around us when we're worried we may forget to do something important.

Do you keep a list so you don't forget to do something? I do, and I love the satisfaction of crossing something off my list—done! But when I didn't get something done on my list, then I would have to make a decision: should I create a new list and re-write what I didn't do or should I keep this list that I currently have but only half the things are done? What about new things, do I add it to my half done to do list or start a separate list?

This was something that I struggled with daily which lead to many pieces of paper with things that I needed to do written on them. I didn't like having multiple pieces of paper that I needed to refer to, and I also didn't like re-writing my to do list every day. Then I discovered... (imagine a trumpet fanfare introducing royalty)... Nozbe. Huh?

Interesting name, I agree. Nozbe is a time management and productivity app designed to help users with tasks. It allows you to add details to your tasks, add deadlines, and manage them within projects (one of my favorite features). The base plan which I use is free. There are so many features in this app, and I know I am just scratching the surface with the features that I use. Nozbe has helped me to get so much out of my head.

In the past, I would have to decide where to write down the tasks that came up during the day. Should I put it in my planner? Should I put it on a post it note? My husband often asked me to do tasks that I didn't want to forget, yet I didn't need to do immediately. I worried that if I didn't write it on my current to do list, I would forget about what he asked me to do since it wasn't right in front of me.

Once I started using Nozbe, this was no longer an issue. I could put the task in the app and assign a due date so I wouldn't forget to do it, and then I didn't have to worry that I would forget to do what he asked me to do. I no longer had to keep re-writing tasks that I hadn't done yet and place them on a new current task list.

As Moms, we have a lot of things that are on our mind at all times. Here are a few things that Moms have running through their heads at any given moment:

- My child's development, health, emotions, doctor visits, sensory needs, feeding issues, school, IEP, buying the next size for shoes and clothes, etc.

- Financial items such as paying the bills, planning for the future, navigating insurance companies and reimbursement, etc.

- Home related things such as cleaning, repairing various items, keeping up with the yard work, maintaining your car, buying groceries and basic necessities, etc.

- Personal stuff such as honoring commitments that you've made, keeping appointments, taking care of your health and well-being, finding time for your spouse, maintaining friendships, etc.

With so much on my mind, I remember feeling so overwhelmed and scattered that I didn't know where to start. I hated that feeling of helplessness that overtook me because I had so much in my head, making it difficult to decide what to do first. When I learned about Nozbe, I wasn't sure if this app would help me since I still would have all these things to do.

The beauty of Nozbe is that it takes all these tasks that are cluttering up your mind and frees you from having to remember and think about them. Once you put these tasks into Nozbe, you don't have to worry about forgetting to do the task or where you wrote it down. All your tasks are in one place.

My friend, Liz, is a busy Mom with two young children. She had so much to do and felt she was moving at warp speed, yet she barely got anything done. I told her about the Nozbe app, and she said she didn't have time to learn another app, but since it was free she downloaded it but didn't look at it.

Another week went by and she decided to test it out. Within minutes of reviewing it, she knew it would change her life. She's been using it every day since. She said it took an hour or two to input all her tasks, but she could feel the difference of having her tasks out of her head and all in one organized place. It felt like a big weight was lifted from her shoulders. She still had the same tasks that she needed to do, but she didn't have to carry these tasks in her head every day wherever she went.

Here's what you can do:

1. If you are interested in downloading the app, download the free version. If you are not interested in an app, then get a notebook and break it into sections by adding tabs to it. However, you should still read through the following steps because you will see the beauty of what Nozbe can do further down.

2. Do a "brain dump." Jot down into your Nozbe "inbox," or your notebook, every task that you have in your head. It can be something that you have to do right away or things that are 6 months in the future. Just get it out of your head.

3. Go through your calendar month by month as it will bring up other tasks that you have floating in your head. Add those tasks to your Nozbe "inbox" or your notebook.

4. You now have a lot of tasks listed, maybe even hundreds of things to do. This is where having the app is awesome. Take a look at these tasks and see if it would make sense to group certain tasks together into a "project." Nozbe gives you five projects to use in their free version. Project categories may be for tasks related to your job, home, child, or even a current project such as planning a birthday party. With Nozbe, you can

take tasks from your inbox and assign them to a project, so that they're grouped together and easy for you to view.

If you don't have Nozbe and are doing this in a notebook, you will not have the luxury of assigning the task to a project for easy reference. If you do want to group it by project, you will need to re-write the task onto a project page in your notebook. The alternative is to think of different projects before you do your brain dump, and then write down your tasks under the project that it relates to. This will slow the process down, but if it's your method of choice, go for it.

5. Next you can assign due dates for your tasks and sort your tasks so that the tasks that are due first are at the top of your task list.

6. To check things off your to do list in Nozbe, you simply tap the spot to mark it as completed, and it gets moved from the top of the list to the bottom where all completed tasks go.

7. Make a habit of checking Nozbe at a set time each day to see what tasks are due and what is coming up.

As part of your nightly routine which we will cover in Chapter 14 Peace of Mind Routine, you will look at your calendar each night and plan for three tasks that you will do the next day. If you complete those three tasks, that's awesome; you can check them off as completed tasks in Nozbe. If you choose to, you know where to go to find more tasks that you can tackle next. If you don't complete the tasks, you don't need to worry about forgetting to do them as they're still in Nozbe.

Even with the best of intentions, there are times when life throws us curves, and we find ourselves juggling too many things at once. This downward spiral leads to mom burnout, which I refer to as "Crazy Lady," causing you to feel so frazzled and on edge at times that you are not thinking straight. Even with all your planning, if things are happening outside of your control and you find yourself falling into Crazy Lady Mode, I have a plan for you...

Chapter 13
If All Else Fails...

*"If you are patient in one moment of anger, you
will avoid one hundred days of sorrow."*
—**Chinese Proverb**

Have you ever had one of those days where everything
that could possibly go wrong went wrong? Perhaps, you
overslept and you're starting the day behind schedule.
You jump out of bed hoping to get dressed before the
kids wake up, but you hear the baby crying. You take care
of the baby and get dressed, but it takes you twice as long
because you are trying to juggle a crying baby and getting
dressed at the same time. Then you make breakfast for
the kids and no one feels like eating. You're looking at the
clock thinking that they need to eat something, or they're
going to be crabby. And you still need to get everyone
dressed before you get out of the door. Just as you have
everyone dressed and are ready to go, your older child
throws a fit about getting his shoes on. You help him

with his shoes, and you're ready to go, but... your baby makes a big poop and now you need to change her and her outfit because it's a big messy one.

The days when I start off feeling scattered and unorganized, I become stressed and reactive to everyone around me. By doing this, I pass on my scattered and unorganized feelings to them, and it becomes a chain reaction. In our house, we call it "the downward spiral," and when you are in the eye of the storm, it is difficult to get out without a plan.

Over the years, I have figured out what triggers these downward spirals. Previous chapters went over what you can do to reduce them. But what if you're in the middle of a downward spiral, what can you do right now? In order to turn things around, you need to put a plan into place now when you're not stressed because when you're at your tipping point, it's harder to think clearly.

Here are a few ideas to help you decompress and bring you down from your tipping point:

1. Bite your tongue—Have you ever said something in a moment of anger or frustration and later been glad that you said those words? I haven't. In fact, I am downright appalled at some of the things that I said on those days when I was losing it and the Crazy Lady in me appeared full swing.

2. Change your environment—Just as a change in environment will often help a child shift out of a

tantrum, this will help you clear your head. Step outside if you can or go to another room.

3. Turn on your favorite tunes—Sometimes it is not possible to leave the room, so instead, put on some headphones and play your favorite music or an interesting podcast to give your mind a break from what is stressing you.

4. Go for a walk—This is a great option if you can't leave your child but need to release some energy. If your child is young enough, put him in a stroller so you can walk at your desired pace and release some of your tension by walking. Even better, you can put in earbuds and listen to your favorite music.

5. Clean away your stress—Start wiping down the tables, sweeping the floors, putting things away. This helps clear stress as it gives you something to focus on but with the added benefit of physical exercise. You will have a cleaner home and have burned off some steam.

6. Meditation—If you have a meditation app on your phone, pull up one of the quick meditations. The Gaiam meditation app on my phone has a "quick break" collection which is comprised of meditations that are 2–4 minutes long. There are meditations for anger, frustration, stress, and so on.

7. Exercise—Do yoga, qigong or other form of exercise.

8. Just breathe—If you are in a situation where you can't leave the room or put on headphones, focus on your breathing. Concentrate on slowing down your breathing: count up as you take a deep breath in, hold your breath, and then count down as you release your breath. Repeat this cycle for a few minutes to help you in the moment.

9. Pick up your hobby—Do something that you love to shift your focus. What do you like to do—knit, read, cook, scrapbook? Go do something that fills you up.

10. Call someone that gets it—Hopefully, you have built your tribe and have someone that you can call that understands what you're going through. Sometimes just having someone that can listen to you for a few minutes helps you to gain a clearer perspective on the situation at hand.

11. Special toy or book—If you rotate your toys and books, you can bring out a much loved item that has been out of rotation to hold your child's interest while you decompress.

Another helpful thing to have in place is a spouse signal for when you feel yourself sliding into Crazy Lady Mode. This should be discussed ahead of time. You can use the time out hand gesture, signal the peace sign, or whatever works for you to let the other person know that you need a set amount of time to decompress.

I recommend setting the amount of time in advance because if you plan on taking 20 minutes to decompress and your spouse is checking in with you at 10 minutes, this could add to your stress level.

If you had a less than stellar parenting moment, be kind and forgive yourself as you are human, and we all make mistakes. Recognize this and do your best to make amends. It will give you closure on this incident rather than leaving you with a nagging guilt for not handling things in a better way.

Now you have a plan in place to minimize your stress level as much as possible given the many things that you are managing each day. Let's move on to how you can gain more time in your day by building solid routines and putting systems into place to streamline your life.

Step 4
R: Routines

"How we eat and sleep and talk to our kids, how we unthinkingly spend our time, attention and money—those are habits that we know exist. And once you understand that habits can change, you have the freedom and the responsibility to remake them. Once you understand that habits can be rebuilt, the power of habit becomes easier to grasp and the only option left is to get to work."
—Charles Duhigg

By clearing away the physical and mental clutter and taking back your email inbox, you have made time in your day to clarify what is important in your life. With fewer things needing your attention, you can more easily manage your daily stress. So now, you need systems in place to know when you will deal with different aspects in your life.

This step of the book covers key things you can do in your life to have more time each day:

1. Peace of Mind Routine

2. Morning and Daily Routine

3. System for Insurance Paperwork

4. Life Skills & Chores

5. Systemize Your Shopping List

Let's keep going with this momentum that you've built—by making little changes each day, which should now be part of your daily life—and create daily routines, giving you even more time each day to do what is most important to you.

Your home is where you spend most of your time, even if you work outside the home; this is where you likely eat most of your meals, sleep, and spend your time. What if you had routines in place which made your life flow better? These routines take the guesswork out of what you need to do each day. Do you actively make the decision every morning, "Should I brush my teeth this morning?" Of course not, you automatically do it without even thinking about it so it is effortless.

Routines are simply habits that we have either fallen into or have been intentional about shaping in our lives. Some routines or habits serve us well such as exercising and eating right. However, there are other habits that either don't serve us or we haven't been intentional about shaping them to serve us.

This is beautifully summed up in the book *Essentialism: The Disciplined Pursuit of Less* by Greg McKeown. "The way of the Essentialist means living by design, not by default. Instead of making choices reactively, the Essentialist deliberately distinguishes the vital few from the trivial many, eliminates the nonessentials, and then removes obstacles so the essential things have clear, smooth passage. In other words, Essentialism is a disciplined, systematic approach for determining where our highest point of contribution lies, then making execution of those things almost effortless." The author touts the importance of routines and clearly shows how the right routines will yield the greatest results.

When we automate things in our lives (through routines and habits), it is amazing how much mental energy we free up by not having to make decisions on the minutia that comes with daily life. First we'll cover a Peace of Mind (bedtime and night time preparation) Routine in order for your Morning Routine to flow smoothly.

The first week or two that you implement the Peace of Mind Routine, you may feel tempted to quit, but I implore you to keep at it for a month. By doing this, the routines that I'm laying out will become habits. Then you will reap the benefits of not having to think about these things so your day will flow better. Moreover, the time it takes to run through your Peace of Mind Routine will decrease significantly as it becomes another effortless routine in your life.

Chapter 14
Peace of Mind Routine

What is the first thing you do after you put your child to sleep each night? Do you collapse on the couch and turn on the TV or scroll through your social media apps? I know the first thing I am tempted to do is sit down at my computer and enjoy some "me time." Time to myself to do whatever I want to do without anyone needing my attention.

I still do this every night, but I do a few things first because I know that once I sit down for my personal time, I'm not going to want to get up and do anything else. I like to have my kitchen and dining room tidied up before the kids are in bed so I don't have to use my "me time" to clean up the kitchen. However, if we've had people over or we had a late dinner and I didn't have a chance to clean before the kids' bedtime, I will clean up as soon as I put them to bed.

Taking 10–15 minutes to clean my kitchen now will save a lot of mental stress the rest of the night and the next morning. Knowing that the kitchen is a mess will bug me so I won't fully enjoy my time to myself, and it will nag at me as I'm falling asleep. I know that the next morning when I go into the kitchen, I will be greeted by a mess if I don't take the time to clean it up the night before.

Thus, I tidy the kitchen and dining room. I prep my coffee maker for the next morning so that all I have to do is press a button. I take my favorite coffee cup out so it's ready as well. I also place my kids' lunch boxes on the counter to remind me to put their lunches (which were prepared earlier in the day) in them the next morning.

Before I sit down for my me time, I do what I usually do to get ready for bed. I take out my contacts, floss and brush my teeth, etc. Whatever I need to do so that once I'm ready to go to sleep, I can just hop into bed, and I don't have to go through a 10 minute process first.

Notice how the time flies when you're relaxing or having fun? It may have felt like five hours to get through bath time, dinner, and the bedtime routine (even though it was really only two hours). Yet, when it comes to your free time, it can feel like you just sat down, but looking at the clock, you realize it's been over 2 hours, and it's time for bed.

There were countless nights I lost track of time and went to bed too late. And it's no wonder, with all of the things that I could only do while my children were asleep, I felt I had to stay up late and get it done. I couldn't work on the insurance paperwork and watch my son at the same time as he could quickly get into something which would make more work for me to clean up. Thus, I stayed up late, but then I would be tired the next day and would tell myself that tonight I would be in bed by 10pm. However, that didn't happen because I didn't do anything different.

By doing some of my bedtime routine earlier, it was easier to get myself to bed on time. I also have a daily reminder in my smartphone, letting me know it's time to go to bed so I don't lose track of time and stay up late.

Before bed, I review what I have scheduled for the next day and write down three things that I plan to accomplish the next day. This could be things I need to do, calls that I need to make, or errands that I need to run. Taking a few minutes to do this the day before is multi-purpose:

1. It reminds me of scheduled events. If I have a dentist appointment on Monday, they typically call to remind me on Friday. However, I have forgotten all about it by Sunday night.

2. It reminds me of anything else that I need to prep for the next day such as packing lunch for the kids, the diaper bag with all the essentials and a snack, etc.

3. It allows me to plan for what I want to get done from my to do list based on what I have scheduled. If I'm going to be at the dentist tomorrow (which is right next to the mall), I plan

on going to the mall and buying that birthday gift I need for next week since I'm right there.

This simple exercise of reviewing what you have planned the next day will help you prepare and welcome the day rather than dread all that you have to do and wonder what you may have forgotten. I find the way that I start my day impacts the way the rest of my day unfolds. Can you think of a morning that you were feeling scattered or upset about something? Did it impact the way that you interacted with your family and anyone else that you came across that morning or even the rest of the day?

On mornings like this, I wish there were a reset button so I could start my day over in a positive way. I do try to shake off any negative impact left over from such mornings. And it makes me value my Peace of Mind and Morning Routine even more.

Here is a summary of what you can do at night to prepare for the next day; do this before you start your "me time" each night:

1. Clean up the kitchen and dining room— Hopefully, this was done before your child's bedtime, but if it wasn't, clean it up now.

2. Prep whatever you need from the kitchen for tomorrow morning—Prep your coffee maker (or hot water kettle if you're a tea drinker) and have your mug ready to go as well. Do your children need their lunch packed before they go off to school? If so, pack their lunch now and put it in

the refrigerator. Or place your children's lunch boxes on the counter so you can quickly place their lunch in them tomorrow. If they're not in school yet, will they need snacks/lunch for an outing if you have plans the next morning? If so, get that together now so tomorrow all you have to do is grab it and go.

3. Get ready for bed—Go through your normal routine such as taking out contacts, brushing your teeth, changing into pajamas, etc.

4. Set reminders—Set an alarm to remind you to go to bed at a certain time each night so you won't get carried away watching a movie or researching on your computer and staying up later than you planned. I have a daily reminder in my phone that says "Go to Bed"; it is set for 30 minutes before I want to go to bed so I have time to wrap up whatever I am doing.

5. Review your schedule—Review what you have scheduled for tomorrow: Is there anything out of the ordinary that you need to have ready? Do you need to bring something to work the next day for a potluck or does your child need to bring something special for school the next day? If the item is non-perishable, leave it by your door so you won't forget to take it the next day. For perishable items, put a sticky note on the door at eye level to remind you to grab it from the refrigerator so you don't leave the house without

it. Everything should be ready now, so that the next morning you just need to grab it and go.

6. Make a plan—Write down 3 things that you plan to do tomorrow. This should be things outside of your normal schedule. It could be things you need to do around the house or with your child, calls that you need to make, or errands that need to be run. If there is anything on your schedule that you can prepare for today, then get that out of the way. For example, if you plan to go to the mall to return something, put the item that you need to return next to your handbag.

If you get through all 3 things on your list the next day—gold star for you, that's awesome! If you want to tackle something else, then select something from your Nozbe list (discussed in Chapter 12 Free Your Mind, Free Your Time), maybe there is a project that you would like to take the next step on.

7. Prep your clothes—Lay out your clothes and accessories for the next morning. This will be one less decision that you have to make and speeds up your morning routine. Depending on where you live, you may want to check the weather forecast for the next day.

If the weather is stable, I will pick out my kids clothes for the week and hang them up in order from Monday through Friday so that I don't have to think about what they're wearing.

I found this especially helpful when my middle child was in second grade and started caring about what she wore to school. I had her select the outfits for the week on Sunday night because if I waited for each weekday morning she would take a while to decide. There would also be clothes all over the floor or a mess in her drawers from rummaging for something to wear; this created a negative start to the day. By having the outfits selected in advance, we avoided the hassle as she could just grab the one in front and get dressed.

If you haven't been doing a bedtime routine or night time prep as I've detailed above, it may seem like I'm asking you to do a lot. However, these things will have to get done anyway, and you will find that if you commit to getting these things done at night when you're not pressed for time, you will have less stress in the morning.

When you put the Peace of Mind Routine into place, the next morning you will feel little bits of happiness every time you go to do something and realize it's already done. You've prepared yourself with these little gifts the night before so this morning you get to reap the benefits. Give yourself a pat on the back for being so prepared; doesn't it feel great?

The wonderful thing about a system like this is that the more that you put into it, the more you will get out of it.

It will give you the momentum to do more with your life because each success that you have reinforces your routine.

Shifting these simple tasks to a different time will allow your morning to proceed a lot more smoothly. This will help the rest of your day flow better as often the way we start our day influences our mindset for the rest of the day. With that said, let's move on to the next chapter to create a morning routine.

Chapter 15
Morning & Daily
Routine

Before you start this chapter, make sure that you have read the previous chapter on the Peace of Mind Routine. This chapter assumes that you have put the previous chapter's routines into place. The Morning Routine in this chapter will not make sense unless you put the Peace of Mind Routine in place first.

Ideally, you will have your Peace of Mind Routine in place for a couple of weeks before you start implementing the Morning Routine. Otherwise, it will be too overwhelming if you implement everything at the same time. You will give up before you have had a chance for the process to become a habit for you.

I suggest while you are waiting two weeks for the Peace of Mind routine to become habitual, start on Chapter 16 System for Insurance Paperwork. This will not interfere with your Peace of Mind Routine as it is not something that you will need to do every day.

With all that said, let's get into your Morning Routine. The key thing to remember in setting up your routine is to be intentional about what you're doing. What do I mean by that? I will give you a framework for setting up a morning routine to help your morning flow well. But unless you are intentional and deliberate about how you set up your routine and execute it, you won't see much benefit.

For example, have you ever gone to a workout class, but your mind was elsewhere? Your body went through the motions of the workout, but your mind was someplace else entirely? When the workout was over, did you feel you had a good workout?

Contrast the scenario I just gave you with going into the workout with the mindset that you're going to get a great workout. With your body and mind fully in this workout, you focus on getting the most out of it. Now, how do you feel afterwards? I'll bet in this scenario you feel you got a much better workout because you intended to have a great workout and were deliberate about it.

You went to the same workout class, spent the same amount of time, but the intentional, deliberate mindset made the difference. This is what I want you to do with this book.

Be intentional and deliberate as you go through each chapter in setting things up in your life and you will reap the greatest benefits.

Let's look at the morning routine that you currently have in place. Do you wake up feeling refreshed and excited to start your day? Do your mornings run smoothly? Is there room for improvement in your morning routine? Let's begin with what you need to do in the morning to start your day.

Let's lay out the basics:

1. Get ready—the time that it takes you to wake up, brush your teeth, do what you need to do before you get dressed such as take a shower, do your hair and make-up etc.

2. Workout—the time that it takes to get your workout in if you do it in the morning.

3. Prepare breakfast—this may be for your entire family or just for your child.

4. Get your child ready—this includes waking, feeding, dressing, etc.

Take a look at what you do on a daily basis in the morning:

- Is there anything that you can prep the night before? If so, add it to your Peace of Mind Checklist.

- Are there any decisions that you make in the morning which you can decide on the night before such as what you are making for breakfast? If you are wondering every morning what you are going to make for breakfast, this slows the flow of your morning.

The days that I don't drive carpool I make a heartier breakfast as I have more time to do that. However, on the days that I drive the morning carpool, I need to have my kids fed, dressed, and loaded into my car by 7:20am. On those mornings, they eat leftovers or my backup plan.

My backup plan is something that they can eat quickly, and that I keep stocked. It is good to have a backup plan for each meal of the day because no matter how prepared you are each day, there will be days that something happens. You will need to adjust for a sick child or if your child is having a difficult day.

- Is there anything you could shift to another time of day? If so, figure out another time of day that you can do it and schedule it. If you don't schedule it, it won't happen.

- Is there anything sidetracking you from making the most of your morning? I.e. social media, email, etc. It may be tempting to go on social media and respond to emails first thing in the morning. Remind yourself that those people are outside of your home, and the most important people in your life are right there in front of you.

When you have a child with autism, you have an endless list of things that need your attention on top of the fact that your child needs extra support. If you have a few spare minutes, you may be tempted to respond to an email or any number of things. In the morning when you're going through your daily routine, resist the urge to do something that is outside of your Morning Routine. This temptation will sidetrack you. Often something you think will take you two minutes, ends up taking five minutes and now you're running late to get your child to speech, OT, school, etc.

The only caveat is if there is something you would like to accomplish in the morning and you intentionally wake up earlier to do it, then you can add it to your routine. For example, in order for me to write this book, I am waking up at 5:15am so I can get an hour of uninterrupted writing time each morning. I do this before the kids wake up as once they are up, I will need to get breakfast started for everyone.

I set my timer so I know what time I need to stop writing, or I will lose track of time and breakfast will start late. I will be running behind and the day will have just begun. When deciding how much time something will take, always allow extra time just in case things don't go as planned.

Speaking of timers, I use timers throughout the day to keep me on track for what I need to do. Here are a few things that I use timers for:

- Once I sit the kids down to breakfast, I tell them how much time they have to eat. When the timer goes off, they need to clear their plates and start brushing their teeth. This is helpful for my middle child as she tends to talk a lot and lose track of time.

- Since my kids have different drop offs and pick-ups during the day, I set the timer so I don't forget when I need to pick them up as I get focused on what I'm doing. This is especially helpful during the summer when their schedule is new, and we don't have an established routine yet.

- I set a timer for my kids when I need them to do a task/chore that they don't want to do, but it will only take them 5 minutes. When I use the timer, my kids turn it into a game to see how much they can get done in the short amount of time.

Let's go over how to determine the timing for your Morning Routine. Your best case scenario for breakfast with your child may be 15 minutes but is this typical? If he normally takes 20 minutes and on hard days takes 25 minutes, then plan for 25 minutes. This way you can have a relaxing stress free morning if he takes a little longer than normal. If you schedule only 15 minutes, you may put unneeded pressure on yourself and your child to finish his meal in 15 minutes.

In order to stick to my routine, I need to stay motivated, keeping in mind the reason I want/need my routines to flow well: 1. It helps me to have a positive mindset for the day, which enables me to start my kids off with a positive mindset to their day. 2. It builds a cushion of time so that I can get where I need to go with ease.

Here's a summary of things to consider as you build your Morning Routine:

1. Be intentional and deliberate about your routine.

2. Prep whatever you can the night before and include it in your Peace of Mind Routine so you can go to sleep knowing you will be fully prepared in the morning.

3. Decide what you are having for breakfast each morning and have a backup plan.

4. Resist checking your email or going onto social media as much as possible.

5. Set a timer to keep you and your child on track.

Now that you have your Morning Routine, let's move on to daily routines. Let's look at the things that have to be done on a daily and weekly basis. These monotonous things offer you the opportunity to set up a routine to make things flow better. In my house, my daily routines consist of doing dishes and laundry, preparing the kids lunches for school the next day, changing the bedsheets, cleaning the house, and preparing dinner.

It feels daunting when you look at all the things you have to do each day, so it helps to create a weekly schedule for recurring tasks. If you schedule your recurring tasks, you won't look at your tasks as a mountain of things you need to do. You will see what you need to get done today. Recurring tasks won't overwhelm you because you've scheduled time for it.

Laundry for us is a daily recurring task since we are a family of five. Everyone's laundry is done once a week with bedsheets and towels done twice a week since they are bulky. We change the bedsheets on Wednesdays, and clean the bathrooms on Thursdays.

Spread the work out and automate the task
so you're not trying to figure out on a daily basis
when something will happen.

As Moms of special needs kids, we have so much on our minds. Setting up a schedule will free you from having to make these decisions on the everyday stuff of life. Debating when we should do something takes away our focus from more important things. I recommend putting up a visual schedule to help you establish this routine.

Take a look at the things you need to do every day and figure out the best time to do it. Be consistent about following your schedule. You will find that these routines will build into habits that you can do quickly.

Loading the dishwasher the night before rather than the next day quickly became a habit I now appreciate. I used to hate doing the dishes even though I have a dishwasher. I felt tired after a meal and didn't feel like loading dishes at that time so I left the dishes in the sink. I would look at it afterwards sitting in the sink and feel drained. Often I left the dishes in the sink overnight and would wake to the sight of dirty dishes that now had food caked on them. I hated that and realized that I had made more work for myself by not loading them the night before.

What's that saying, 'you don't know what you've got until it's gone?' I learned that lesson when my dishwasher gave out on me. This meant researching the different brands, ordering it, and waiting for my new dishwasher to arrive. In the meantime, I had to wash dishes by hand, and boy, did I appreciate my dishwasher now.

My mindset went from looking at loading the dishwasher as a chore to being grateful that I have a working dishwasher. Now I put the dishes into the dishwasher as soon as I get up from the table. It doesn't take long, my sink is empty, and my mind is clear from the nagging voice telling me I have a huge mess of dishes waiting for me. I put on my favorite music while cleaning, and the time flies by and my kitchen is clean.

Find a time that works best for your everyday tasks. This works well for fun things too such as things you do with your kids: reading, sensory play, outside time, etc. Investing the time to look at your schedule and figure out when it makes sense to do things will save you a lot of mental energy.

Initially, you will need the schedules and checklists to remember everything you need to do. In time, your scheduled tasks will become a routine, and you will find more positive habits to help your day flow well.

If you have school aged children, you may find you need the schedules and checklists again when you return from summer or winter break. These breaks take us out of our daily routine, and often, we need the reminders to get back into our good habits and routines.

Here's a summary of things to consider as you build your daily routines:

1. Make a list of recurring things you do on a daily basis such as doing the dishes and laundry, preparing the kids' lunches for school the next day, cleaning the house, and preparing dinner.

2. Figure out the best time to do this and consistently do it at that time.

3. Put the schedule where you can see it or write it into your calendar for a couple of weeks until this becomes routine for you.

As Moms, a lot of things need our attention. I hope that putting routines in place will help you have more time to do the meaningful things in your life rather than worrying about the mundane.

We have covered the framework for setting up a Morning and Daily Routine. It will take a couple of weeks for this to become a habit for you, but once it does, you will feel the shift in your mindset. Your mind won't constantly try to figure out what you have to do and when you have to do it. You will just know.

You now have a great framework for establishing your household routines. Next, I want to show you a great system for handling therapy bills, insurance forms, tracking reimbursement and more. You will have a place for everything and know where you are with each invoice that you've paid.

Chapter 16
System for Insurance Paperwork

You should have your Peace of Mind Routine in place now helping you start your day in a positive way. In this chapter, I will show you a system for handling your insurance paperwork. The forms, reports, and invoices can lead to piles of paper everywhere. These important papers relate to insurance reimbursement that you want to stay on top of to submit your claims on time.

Papers are constantly entering your home whether through the mail, work, or your child's school or therapist. If you don't have a system for handling the incoming flow of paperwork, then it tends to pile up. You may have papers you intend to sift through when you have time. Maybe, you even put the important ones on top of the pile. This was my system for dealing with papers that entered my home. I say system, but really it was lack of a system that led to so many piles.

I did have one thing that significantly reduced my paper piles. Every day when the mail came into the house, I would immediately throw the junk mail into the recycle bin. Any bills that required payment went straight to my checkbook to be reviewed and paid when I was ready to do that. Any checks that came in the mail also went straight to my checkbook so that I had everything in one place when I was ready to deposit them.

It was the insurance paperwork that loomed over my head. There were so many things coming to me at different times. I had paid invoices for my child's therapy, claim forms that I needed to complete and submit, rejected claims that came back from the insurance company which I would have to contest, and there were the paid claims and explanation of benefits that I needed to reconcile.

Every bill was in a different part of the cycle, and I needed a simple system for tracking where it was in the cycle. Had I submitted it for insurance yet? Did I get reimbursed yet? Did this claim get rejected and need to be contested?

I wanted an easy to maintain system that I could see at a glance where I was in the process. I also wanted to ensure that insurance paperwork didn't get lost in the sea of other household paperwork (bills, forms, mail, and kids' schoolwork).

Let me step back and first go over the process for paying a bill, especially for therapists that you see multiple times a week. Therapy is expensive, and those therapy visits add up fast so you want to ensure that you're only billed for appointments you kept. Maybe you took a planned vacation or the therapist was sick, so be sure that you were not billed for those sessions. Here's what I do to track therapy sessions, which has the added benefit of tracking medical miles for therapists that I see outside of my home:

1. Write down all therapy appointments in your calendar, including the time and therapist's initials. Do this for the entire month.

2. At the end of each day, review your calendar and put a check mark next to each session your child attended. If the session was cancelled, cross out the session (don't erase it!). Next to it, write down why the session was cancelled such as "T sick" or "A vac" so you know why the session was cancelled (sick, vacation, etc.) and who cancelled the session (you or the therapist). This will be helpful when you are reviewing the invoice as it is difficult to remember if and why a session was cancelled a month ago.

3. When it comes time to pay your therapy bill, review your calendar and check that it matches your bill. If it doesn't, contact your provider to get a revised invoice before you pay it.

Now let's go over how to set up a System for Insurance Paperwork:

1. Create an accordion file for insurance reimbursement; this accordion file will simplify the insurance reimbursement process for you and keep all your insurance paperwork together. You can buy a basic letter size accordion file from places such as Target, Walgreens, or any office supply store. Make sure to get one that has at least 8 tabs inside. The one I use has lasted for years; I've seen them for $5 so it is a minimal investment to stay organized.

2. Once you have your accordion file, set up the following tabs:

   a. Paid Invoices

   b. New Insurance Communication

   c. Submitted to Insurance

   d. Contest Claim

   e. Update Schedule

   f. Claim Forms

   g. Labels & Envelopes

   h. File

3. Stock your newly set up accordion file. Complete the basic information for your family on a claim form (name, address, insurance id info). Make copies of this form so you don't have to re-write this information every time that you need to submit a claim, and place those copies in the Claim Forms section.

4. If you know how to create address labels, I suggest making them to simplify the process if you have a lot of claims. I use labels from Avery as their label templates are in my computer which made it easy for me to do. Use return address labels or a self-inking stamp (if you have one) for your home address. Prep the envelopes so they are ready to go with your insurance company mailing address as well as your return address. You may want to keep a book of stamps in this section as well.

5. Fill in the other tabs:

   a. Place all invoices that you have already paid but have not submitted to insurance in the first tab labeled "Paid Invoices."

   b. Place new communication from your insurance company in the tab marked "New Insurance Communication." When you receive paperwork from the insurance company, place it in this tab so you don't misplace it. When you are ready to do your next round of insurance claims, you will have everything together, and you won't have to go looking for it.

c. Place copies of invoices that have been submitted to your insurance company but have not been reimbursed yet under the tab "Submitted to Insurance."

d. Once you have received reimbursement from your insurance company, match it with the copy of the invoice that you submitted (which was under the "Submitted to Insurance" section). Staple this together and place it in the "Update Schedule" section.

e. You may receive a claim denial from your insurance company with a processing claim error. Place the claim denial from the insurance company along with the applicable invoice under "Contest Claim."

6. Pick a date and time once a month to process all your current claims and follow up on any claims that you need to contest with your insurance company. As you pay invoices and new communication arrives from your insurance company, place it in your accordion file. Don't worry about losing the paperwork or when you're going to process it as you already have a time scheduled to process claims.

Check your insurance company policy for the timing requirements on claims. Some insurance companies may give you up to 6 months and others may give you only 90 days for an out of network claim. Make sure you understand your insurance company's claim reimbursement policy so you know the deadline for submitting claims.

7. When it is time to go through your insurance paperwork, download from my website (www.AutismMomMindset.com/downloads) and follow the "Insurance Reimbursement Process" flow chart illustrating how the paperwork travels through your system. If you are being denied for claims that should be covered by your insurance policy and follow up with your insurance company has not helped, you may want to check out the Mental Health & Autism Insurance Project (www.autismhealthinsurance.org). Once you have processed all your paperwork for the month, proceed to the update schedule step.

8. Create a Medical Expenses Schedule. This is a dual purpose spreadsheet for tracking reimbursement as well as tracking medical expenses for tax purposes. Group expenses by type and vendor so you can see which vendor you have filed claims for and which ones you have received reimbursement.

Check to see if you are above the medical expense threshold for IRS purposes. If you are, you can use this spreadsheet as a starting point for doing your taxes. You may be interested in tracking your medical miles as well.

9. If you are above the medical expenses threshold for IRS purposes, you may want to create a Medical Miles spreadsheet. Calculate the miles driven for anything that qualifies as medical expense under the IRS guidelines. Use this spreadsheet as well as the monthly invoice for each vendor to calculate how many times you travelled for medical reasons.

If you are tracking therapy sessions in your calendar with a check mark, you can go through each month and add up the check marks for each vendor. Add them to your Medical Miles spreadsheet. This is a good way to ensure you captured all your miles.

Once you have your system in place, I hope that the insurance reimbursement process and keeping track of it all is weighing less on your mind. Now, are you ready to cover something that will pay you back for your time investment over and over again for years to come? Let's do this!

INSURANCE REIMBURSEMENT PROCESS

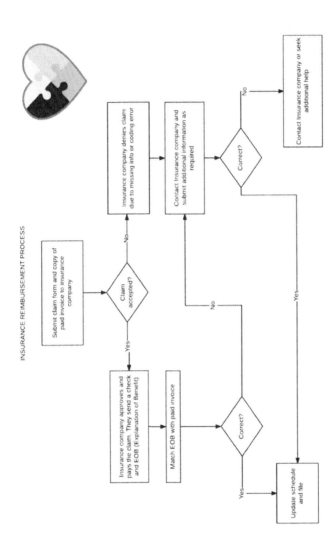

```
Submit claim form and copy of
paid invoice to insurance
company
            │
            ▼
      ┌─────────────┐
      │    Claim    │──── No ──►┌──────────────────────┐
      │  accepted?  │           │ Insurance company    │
      └─────────────┘           │ denies claim due to  │
            │                   │ missing info or      │
           Yes                  │ coding error         │
            │                   └──────────────────────┘
            ▼                              │
┌──────────────────────────┐              ▼
│ Insurance company         │   ┌──────────────────────┐
│ approves and pays the     │   │ Contact insurance    │
│ claim. They send a check  │   │ company and submit   │
│ and EOB (Explanation of   │   │ additional           │
│ Benefit)                  │   │ information as       │
└──────────────────────────┘   │ required             │
            │                   └──────────────────────┘
            ▼                              │
┌──────────────────────────┐              ▼
│ Match EOB with paid       │        ┌──────────┐
│ invoice                   │        │ Correct? │── No ──►┌────────────────────┐
└──────────────────────────┘        └──────────┘         │ Contact insurance  │
            │                             │               │ company or seek    │
            ▼                            Yes              │ additional help    │
      ┌──────────┐                        │               └────────────────────┘
      │ Correct? │── No ───────────────────┘
      └──────────┘
            │
           Yes
            │
            ▼
┌──────────────────┐
│ Update schedule  │◄── Yes
│ and file         │
└──────────────────┘
```

Chapter 17
Life Skills & Chores

When my son was about 8 years old, I was given advice from a Mom with an adult son with autism. She advised me to look ahead and determine what I wanted my son to do independently as an adult. She said parents focus on helping their children with so many things. Yet, we forget that we need to start teaching them steps towards independence now as this process takes time.

She spoke from experience when she said that the years will fly by and if you don't start training your child now, he will not be able to do things independently down the road. She was right; it has been five years since I heard her advice and my son is now a teenager. That sage advice motivates me to teach my son skills that will help him to lead as independent a life that is possible for him.

Teaching your children how to do chores is a double win: they learn skills that will benefit them at home and in school for the rest of their lives, and they will be helping around the house, lessening your load. Doesn't that sound wonderful? Think back to when you went off to college, do you remember meeting someone that didn't know how to do anything? Things like washing clothes, cooking a meal, and/or cleaning the bathroom?

Now is the time to start thinking about what your child can do around the house to learn these independent life skills. Taking the time to train him today will pay off many times over through the years. Look at what he can do and show him in small steps how to do it.

One of the first chores parents teach their children is how to put away their toys. The most important thing to remember when teaching your child anything is to have minimal expectations when you train him since he probably won't do it exactly as you wish the first time. Keep your expectations in check, so you aren't sorely disappointed.

Kids with autism or without autism are still kids and ALL kids need to be taught how to do things. It takes time and patience for them to learn how to do things on their own. You will need to model what you need them to do many times. Start with the mindset that this is not something that your child will learn right away. You are starting to train him now because eventually he will learn this skill.

Give yourself plenty of extra time for training. For instance if you're teaching something that takes one minute to complete, give yourself five minutes to train your child. You should only start training when you have plenty of time and are not rushed to go and do something else. This puts extra pressure on you and your child if you are trying to train him but have to be out of the house in three minutes to get to an appointment.

Let's go over an example of training your child to pick up his toys using a positive tone of voice and minimal explanation:

1. Ask your child if he is "all done" with the toys.

2. Tell him it's "clean up time."

3. Show him how to put his toys away. Hopefully, he is playing with something that has multiple parts so you can put some away first to model what "clean up time" looks like. Have him put at least one part away and count that as a success. If your child is resistant, try to find a fun way to encourage him to do it such as singing the clean-up song or doing a little dance while you clean up.

4. Tell him that he did a great job cleaning up.

Your child may not learn this the first time you teach him or even the fifth time, but give yourself a month and see what progress your child has made. If you model each day how to do something and praise your child when he does it, you should see your child progress over time.

Celebrate those small wins, and they will build over time. Consider adding his progress to your gratitude journal covered in Chapter 9 Give Thanks. This is helpful for when you are struggling to teach your child something new. You can look back on something that you struggled with teaching him and see the progress your child has made.

To get you started, here are some ideas of tasks your child may be able to do. Some of these tasks are chores and some are life skills. Select only one new thing to teach your child at a time. Once your child can complete a task independently and it has become a part of his daily routine, then move on to training him on a new task.

- Clean up toys.

- Put his dirty clothes in the hamper.

- Put his towel in the hamper.

- Put his shoes into the shoe cabinet.

- Take his dish to the kitchen after a meal, throw excess food into the trash, and put his plate on the counter (or in the sink if he is tall enough).

- Get out the silverware or cups.

- Teach him where things are so he can get it for you. (Show your child where you keep your utensils and explain what they are so he can get a spoon or fork if you ask him to.)

- Set the table.

- Wipe down the table after a meal.

- Use a dustpan and hand broom to sweep under the table to pick up crumbs.

Also keep in mind that this is a child, and he will forget to do things, a gentle reminder or a visual schedule may help him remember. Taking the time to teach him the simplest things will make your life a lot easier. Another wonderful benefit is the boost to your child's self-esteem when he learns how to do something on his own.

When you know that your child can do something but isn't motivated to do it, you can use music to get him going. There are times when I don't feel like cleaning up (kitchen, my closet, shall I go on?). But I turn on my favorite tunes and somehow whatever I need to clean seems like less of a chore.

Once you have trained your child, it is helpful to have a list of things that your child can do on a daily basis as part of his household responsibility. To help you out, post a clear visual schedule outlining his daily tasks for the week in a prominent spot in your home. Eventually, when you want your child to do his chore, you don't have to nag him just tell him to check his schedule.

Peace of Mind Routine in place? Yup! Morning and Daily Routine in place? Of course! System for Insurance Paperwork in place? You betcha! Life Skills & Chores in progress? Definitely! Ready to move on to our last chapter on routines? Absolutely!

Chapter 18
Systemize Your
Shopping List

In the last chapter, I went over how to train your kids to help with chores and learn life skills. Teaching them these valuable skills will help them in many areas of their life and will free up your time so that you don't have to do everything for them. Another great way to save you time is to run less errands by automating what you buy often.

Minimizing the need to run errands saves me a lot of time. I reduce the amount of errands that I have to run and order what I can online. By doing this, I don't need to gather my kids, load them in the car, drive to the store, shop for what we need, load them back into the car, and drive home. This saves me time, energy, and gas.

A few years ago, I made a list of the items that I buy often. Toiletry items such as shampoo, conditioner, sunscreen, etc. as well as supplements that my family takes. I researched prices and found there were a few places that sold the items I purchase frequently at a discounted price.

Prior to this, I was spending a lot of time comparing prices on websites to find the best price. Looking back, I wasted a lot of my time doing this just to save a small amount.

I have shifted my focus to purchasing my everyday items from a few retailers that offer overall savings. This saves me time since I don't need to go bargain hunting on different websites. Additionally, I feel comfortable with these retailers' customer service, which may not be the case with new retailers I check out just to save a few cents.

Below I have listed the retailers that I shop with: businesses with free shipping and no subscription fees and businesses that charge a subscription fee.

No Subscription Fee Business with Free Shipping:

iHerb.com sells a large selection of natural products. I like this company because they have a low threshold for free shipping ($20 for shipments in the United States), great customer service, eco-friendly initiatives and a large selection of natural products. They sell a lot of products that my family uses so I don't have to order from different websites. They have a rewards program which results in greater savings.

As of January 2016, their latest loyalty program gives customers a loyalty credit for every order placed and shipped. The credit is for 10% off the order value, excluding shipping charges if any, and can be used toward your next order. You have 60 days to use the credit before it expires. This is their policy at the time of writing; please check iHerb's website to see their current rewards program.

If you are interested in using my affiliate coupon code, you will get $5 off your first order, and I will get a discount as well. My code is: COB393. Please note that it is the letter "O" and not a zero. You can also access my web page to see my reviews of my favorite items. (www.iherb.com/me/AutismMom)

I order most of my toiletries and some of my supplements from this website. I purchase natural products as much as possible. Environmental Working Group's Cosmetic Database (www.CosmeticsDatabase.com) provides safety ratings for various beauty products as well as sunscreen and hundreds of other products.

Once I find something that I like at iHerb, I add it to my wish list so I don't have to search for it the next time I want to buy the item. This makes shopping for toiletry items so simple as they are just a few clicks away: I just select the items I need from my wish list, and they are on their way.

Curbside is a free service which simplifies running errands. Simply order and pay through their app on your phone or computer, and they will let you know when your order is ready for pick up. Swing by the store, and they will place your bag in your car for you. This works well if you have a napping child or just don't want to take the extra time to unload your child in and out of the car and stand in line.

According to their website, Curbside is "available at hundreds of CVS locations across Northern California, Atlanta Metropolitan Area, and the Greater Charlotte Metro Area, select Shopping Centers, Sephora, Levi's and more." I find this service especially useful during the holiday season when lines are longer and parking is limited. Check out their website for more information.

Keep in mind when Curbside opens at a new store, they may not have the drive through set up right away. This means that until they are fully set up, you may have to walk in to get your purchases from a pick up counter. Once they are fully onboard with a store, the process is seamless and you just drive up and get your purchases.

Subscription Fee Business with Free Shipping:

Amazon Family, according to Amazon's website, "provides Prime members exclusive family-oriented offers, coupons, age-based recommendations, 20% off diaper subscriptions and a 15% Baby Registry completion discount."

Currently, the cost of an Amazon Prime membership is $99 per year. There are many benefits included with this annual membership such as free two-day shipping, prime video (unlimited instant streaming of thousands of movies and TV shows), prime music (unlimited, ad-free access to over a million songs and thousands of playlists and stations), prime photos (unlimited photo storage in Amazon cloud drive) and more. Check out their website for more information.

I use their subscribe & save program every month and have a standing order for items that my family consumes regularly. By ordering five items in the subscribe & save category, all items qualify for 15% off. Some things that I order are anti-bacterial wipes, dish washing liquid, protein bars, etc. This program is great if you still need diapers and wipes as they have a good selection at a discount and free delivery (since subscribe & save items get free prime delivery).

Google Shopping Express is a paid service which allows you to get same day, next day, or two day delivery of items from national and local stores. My favorites are Costco, Target, Whole Foods and a local toy store, but they have a large list of stores to shop from. I also like that I can shop for an item and see the price of this item across the different stores.

A Google Express membership is $10/month or $95/year. If you prefer not to get a membership, non-member delivery starts at $4.99 per store. Check out their website for more information. They also allow you to link your membership cards from the places that you shop so you still get your rewards points from those stores. If you would like to get $15 off your first order, please use my referral code which is: 36VSYS5EC.

This service is wonderful for bulky items as it is delivered right to your doorstep. Things like dog or cat food, bottled water, laundry detergent, toilet paper, etc. You don't have to worry about juggling your child and carrying something heavy. Also it saves me the trouble of going to places that have long lines such as Costco. They don't have every single item from a vendor available, but there is a lot to choose from.

As an Autism Mom, I have therapists coming and going from my home on a daily basis. When my son was first diagnosed, I took him to his different therapies and groups while juggling my younger daughter's nap schedule and feedings. I didn't have the luxury of using some of these services because I didn't know about them or they didn't exist back in 2006.

If I needed to buy something, I had to figure out when I could go and how I would manage my baby daughter and son at the same time. My son has a history of wandering off, and if he saw something water related, he may bolt towards it with no regard for his personal safety.

I used to stress myself out worrying about when and how I was going to buy things, but now with these shopping options, I no longer have that burden to deal with. This saves me time, energy, and gas, which is a great winning combination.

Step R of the H.E.A.R.T. Method asked you to put routines in place, allowing you more time to focus on your priorities. You should now have a Peace of Mind Routine, Morning Routine, and Daily Routine as well as a system to manage those piling insurance claims, a process for training your kids on life skills and chores, and several options for systemizing your shopping.

With all this accomplished, it's time for the final step of the H.E.A.R.T. Method. The final step is T for Thrive. I wish that Moms would start their self-care earlier on in this journey. Yet, every Mom I know, including myself, wouldn't consider doing this until she had other things in place for her family first. Now that you have those things in place, let's move on to the final step.

Step 5
T: Thrive

"When you recover or discover something that nourishes your soul and brings joy, care enough about yourself to make room for it in your life."
—*Jean Shinoda Bolen*

In this step, I would like to shed a light on self-care. Lately, the media has turned self-care into a buzz word. I used to look at self-care as a luxury, thinking that I didn't have time to pamper myself. I thought my son's needs and behaviors needed my attention more than anything else. If I took time for myself, I was giving up valuable time that could be spent helping him.

This self-less mentality has a price: for me, it meant that I was frazzled all the time. I was tired, cranky, and went into Crazy Lady Mode at random times due to fatigue, and looking back, due to resentment. My logical mind knew that it wasn't my son's fault that he had sensory issues and behaviors. However, a lack of self-care, exhaustion, and an ever growing to do list clouded my judgment.

In the first four steps, I covered how to H: Heal by Learning, E: Energize, A: Anticipate and R: put Routines in place. These are all critical areas that I think every autism Mom should explore. The next few chapters are the areas that will truly help you and your family enrich your life and grow.

Chapter 19
Feed Your Soul

You have an IEP binder, night time and morning routines in place, and a system for your insurance paperwork. Now that you have a bit of breathing room in your life to do something you love, the question is… what do you love to do? I was overwhelmed with all things autism when my son was diagnosed. It took me years to figure out a system and routines to allow me to have time for me.

I hope that by reading this book and putting systems and routines in place, you can start focusing on yourself a lot sooner than I did. As the primary caregiver of a special needs child, an aging parent or even a baby, you hear a lot about self-care.

When you were expecting your first child, I'm sure you heard from a lot of moms that you should take care of yourself. You should sleep when the baby sleeps, etc. They knew what you didn't know yet: being the primary caregiver of a baby is exhausting. You have demands placed on you 24/7, and you need to take care of yourself to be able to take care of your baby.

When a baby grows and transitions out of the toddler stage, his independence grows and his demands on his mom decrease. Mom will have more free time to do the things she loves. A child with autism transitions out of the toddler stage but his sense of independence does not grow. Instead, there are even more demands on his mom.

The "autism mom" now needs to learn a whole new world, a world that comes with its own:

- Vocabulary and acronyms

- Doctors and therapists

- Therapies and best practices

- Conflicting points of view

- Theories on how to advocate for her child

- And a boatload of paperwork

While the typical mom is now reaping the benefits of raising a baby through toddlerhood, the autism mom's workload is about to increase exponentially. She will be busy navigating this new world and juggling more demands on her time. She will need to find her new normal.

Looking back at this phase of my life, it was ten years ago, I remember how devastated and lost I felt. I remember the grief and the fear I felt for my son's future. Every night I went to sleep feeling stressed and overwhelmed, and I woke up feeling such sadness. I wanted to figure out how to help my son and myself. There simply wasn't enough time to help myself as every waking minute was focused on doing something related to my son.

I hope that by implementing the various suggestions, routines, and systems in this book, you will be able to find a new normal for yourself. And that your new normal will involve self-care, so you don't have to wait years to figure things out.

It sounds counter intuitive to take time for yourself when you have a million things needing your attention. Yet, it is through actually taking this time to pause and do something for yourself that you will feel refreshed, enabling you to give 100% to what you need to do.

If you don't make your health a priority, you may have consequences to deal with on top of your mountain of responsibilities. I've experienced this myself with neglecting my own health needs, a lack of exercise, and poor eating habits.

A little self-care will go a long way and your mind and body will reap the benefits with renewed energy and enthusiasm. This in turn will enable you to function at a higher level and open the door to accomplishing more each day.

Let's dive into what feeds your soul, what brings you joy? What did you enjoy doing before you entered the world of autism? If you can't think of anything, look back into your childhood and reflect on what you loved doing. Back then you had a lot of free time to do what you loved. Did you like riding your bike? Roller skating? Swimming? Hiking? Baking? Playing the guitar?

I loved reading and journaling when I was a kid and remember my Dad asking me why I was crying while I was reading a novel and I responded "Because it's so good!" Yet I hadn't read a book in years and months would go by without a journal entry. At the time I felt like it would be selfish to spend time on myself when I had so much to do. It's no wonder I was so miserable, stressed, and tired.

I now enjoy listening to audio books and my children love it as well. It doesn't take up any time as we're listening in the car. It has opened opportunities to discuss life's lessons that come up in the stories and I enjoy children's literature. I have read more books in the last 3 years than I had in the 7 years prior to that. When I hear of a book that sounds interesting, I add it a list that I keep in my phone so that I always have a go to reading list.

I also started journaling again. I had filled many journals over the years, from the time that I was six years old until the time that my son was diagnosed. And then everything stopped. But, I wanted my daughter to have a special journal for her with my thoughts and memories of her growing up, so I started up again.

Since I was so overwhelmed with all that I had to do related to my son, this journal was my small way of doing something for her that she could look back on. I wrote in it sporadically but tried to write down things that she was into at the time—songs that she loved, games that she played, even our special bedtime routine.

With the busyness of life propelling forward, suddenly she wasn't a little toddler anymore. She was in school and like any child, she had good days and bad days. This special journal that I had set aside was something I saved for those bad days. I would read her a journal entry and she would laugh and try to remember the event, but she couldn't because she was only two or three at the time. She loves going back to *her* special journal, I wish I had written more in it at the time, but I'm glad that I have something special for her.

Now that I have my gratitude journal and the 5 Minute Journal, I have a lot more beautiful memories recorded for our family. Every time that I took a few minutes to do that, I felt good doing something that brings me joy.

I have also carved out time each week to exercise—some of it is with my kids as I take them on walks or bike and scooter rides and some are on my own. A fun way to get some exercise in is GoNoodle; it is a free website that has hundreds of short videos intended to get kids moving. According to their website, "GoNoodle turns movement into a game and makes it easy to be active, the kid way— silly, energetic, playful, and fun. Just press play on hundreds of custom-created videos and get kids running, jumping, dancing, stretching, and practicing moments of mindfulness."

GoNoodle's website is easy to maneuver so you can search for videos by categories such as guided dancing, free movement, stretching, etc. If the weather isn't great and we need to do something inside, we will put on a few of these videos and have a great time moving and laughing as we do the motions. The beauty of this is that moving my body makes me feel great (mentally and physically) and sets a great example for my kids. They see the importance that I place on exercise, realize that it's fun, and have now adopted this philosophy for themselves.

Let's recap:

- Think about what brings you joy; what feeds your soul? Reach back into your childhood memories if you need to.

- Figure out a way to start doing this, even if it's just once a week. If it's something that you will need to purchase such as a bike or a guitar, then make that happen. If it's something that you need to sign up for like drama class or cooking lessons, get moving on that. There are inexpensive ways you can buy something second hand or take a class through your community center.

  Here's a list of things to spark ideas for you:

  ▪ Play an instrument

- Read a book

- Journal

- Cook or bake

- Hike, swim, skate, bike, Zumba

- Scrapbook or stamping homemade cards

- Dance

- Paint, sketch, pottery work, photography

- Jewelry making, sew, quilt, knit

- Volunteer work

- Go and do what you love and see how you feel. Are you feeling energized? Are you able to give more to your family because you have a higher sense of personal fulfillment? I hope so!

Don't get me wrong, you still have a lot to manage as an autism mom. Finding something that brings you joy won't make all those things go away, but it does fill you up when there are so many demands on you.

I don't want you to come down from the high of doing something that you love just yet so let's discuss the next area that will add some joy into your life.

Chapter 20
Your Environment

Figuring out and actually doing something that brings you joy is incredible. Even if you are only able to squeeze in 15 minutes a day to play the piano, do some sketch work, or dive into a book, you will start to reap the benefits of doing something for you.

Let's go over the things that will have an impact on you every day—your environment. Your environment has a strong impact on your happiness. You tend to spend the majority of your day in the same places whether in your home, office, or even car.

In Chapter 11 Zen Zone = Happy Home, we went over the importance of clearing out the clutter in your life. Assuming you have done this already, I want to go over a few things that you can do to enhance your environment.

You want to surround yourself with things that bring you happiness. However, since your environment is personal to you, I don't know what evokes happiness in your heart when you look around you; thus, I will share some of the things that make me smile every time I look at them, which may give you some inspiration.

I was first introduced to this concept by my husband many years ago when we were students. He would talk about his lucky pencil, and then there was his lucky ring, and his lucky mug. I asked him how many "lucky" things he had. He said he didn't know, he just liked his favorite things around him and he called them "lucky."

At the time, I thought it was just this fun thing that he did. But research shows that activating good luck superstitions through good luck charms can improve performance. For me, surrounding myself with lucky things brings a little bit of happiness into my life each time I glance at or use the item.

I'm sitting in my office right now and a few of my lucky things are right in my field of vision. My lucky pink mug—I have 2 lucky mugs (a pink one in the morning that I drink my coffee in and a mama bear cup in the afternoon for my tea). I see a beautiful orchid in a pretty pot and a picture of my Grandma and me from almost 20 years ago.

My eyes can't help but notice these simple everyday items; they are special and meaningful to me. I may not stop and reflect on them every time I come into contact with them, but there have been many times that I was trying to figure something out, and when I looked at one of my lucky things, it brought me a sense of peace. It's a reminder of a wonderful person or shared experience.

As an Autism Mom, there are times in my life when I feel so completely overwhelmed with my child, myself and my life. There are so many demands on me all at once that I literally don't know where to start. Having these special things scattered throughout my day brings me peace and grounds me when I'm in the midst of all the chaos.

The pink mug reminds me of a fun afternoon with my best friend. I found it when we had gone shopping and out to eat.

The orchid I bought at the farmer's market for $7, and it is a beautiful reminder of my family's tradition: going to the farmer's market.

The picture of my Grandma and me is a spontaneous picture my cousin took at my brother's wedding. My Grandma passed away a couple of years later, but at the time this picture was taken, she was 94 years old and doing great. It is framed, and the only photograph that I have on my desk. When I look at it, I'm reminded of my grandma, who found pleasure in her daily rituals with her positive and grateful attitude. She exercised every morning, danced at the senior center, enjoyed eating papaya at 3:00pm, and did her evening stretches before going to bed each night.

Lucky items don't have to be something that cost you a lot of money, it can be things that you have, but they are tucked away so you don't see them every day. If it is something that brings you happiness when you see it or use it, take it out and make the item part of your daily life. As you are deciding which items to use in your everyday life, be mindful of your family and other people in your home. Use your discretion on whether you should display a fragile figurine on your desk as curious hands may want to touch it.

Here are a few of my favorite things (I can't help hearing Julie Andrews beautiful voice in my head):

- Pink mug & mama bear mug

- Orchid

- Framed photo of my Grandma and me.

- Mechanical pencil that I used throughout college and forgot about. I found it years ago and placed it on my desk so I can use it daily.

- Special artwork that my kids made for me.

- Earrings—I have several lucky earrings that are from various people that I love.

- Watch

- Decorative wedding plate displayed in the kitchen.

- Pretty notebooks

- Pencil case—its bright yellow and fun. I keep it in my purse as it makes me happy every time I look at it.

The lucky items I listed above are all visual things; however, music can also be a lucky thing impacting your environment. How often do you listen to your favorite music? Music is so personal; a song can touch your heart and really lift your spirit. It can energize and inspire you.

I have my favorite music downloaded on my phone and listen to it when I'm cleaning the kitchen or doing other chores around the house. I also use music to shift the mood of my children. When I'm driving my kids somewhere and I can tell they are tired or grumpy, I have my daughter use my phone, and she becomes the backseat DJ. She puts on music that they like, and everyone's spirit and energy level rises with the music that they enjoy.

In Chapter 17 Life Skills & Chores, I discussed how I use music in my environment to motivate my kids to do their chores. Another way that I have used music is to drown out undesirable noises. When my son was younger, he made a lot of noises and echolalia (repeating sentences over and over). It used to drive me crazy hearing this all day.

Rationally, I knew that my son couldn't help making these noises; he wasn't trying to torment me. But I must admit, hearing these noises day after day, every day for months... I started going a little crazy. We were working on different strategies to reduce this but change takes time. In the meantime, putting on music helped to block out some of the noise. It also helped my son as he enjoys music and would often choose to stop and listen to it rather than repeat the same thing over and over.

If you have Amazon Prime, you can listen to Amazon Prime Music which includes access to over a million songs and hundreds of playlists for free. It's included in your Prime membership and works like other subscription music providers such as Spotify. There are no commercials to listen to, and you can choose to give a song a thumbs down and skip it.

I love that this service is part of my Amazon Prime membership as I use it daily. It has introduced me to a lot of music that I never would have discovered without it. In fact, I am listening to their Classical Focus Prime Station right now because I like music in the background when I'm writing. I need it to be instrumental, or I will start singing along. My daughter listens to it when she is doing her homework.

Through this Classical Focus Prime Station, I have some beautiful classical pieces which I love to listen to. It's wonderful how listening to music that you love can completely shift your mood. The app makes it easy to download the songs that you love so you can take it with you and you don't have to be connected to the internet.

Sprinkle your lucky things throughout your day and savor the joy that fills your heart and comes from the simple things in your life. These simple things along with your favorite music will elevate your environment. Once you have your music downloaded, where do you want to go? I can think of several great places to go to with or without your child to round out this final section on taking care of yourself.

Chapter 21
Get Out & Remember
Who You Are

Are you feeling happy from playing your favorite tunes? Are you doing some things with more ease and a skip in your step? I hope you are surrounding yourself with beautiful music to elevate your spirit.

For our final chapter on self-care, I would like to discuss the importance of getting outside. I mean this in the broadest sense possible—go outside, even if it's just your backyard. Sometimes with all of the signs of autism everywhere you look—paperwork, sensory toys, insurance reimbursement, IEP binder, etc.,—it helps to just get out of the house. Autism may be on your mind constantly, but it doesn't need to be everywhere you look as well.

Step outside for a walk or a bike ride. When the weather is nice, we like to go for a family walk. It's nice to go for a walk in the afternoon or after dinner. When our two older children were younger, they liked to ride their scooters. You can also read with your child in the backyard instead of in the house. Just make sure you spend some time outside. If you are able to, then go to the park, the beach, or to the movies. If you are nervous about your child standing out and being bullied by other kids, meet up with other special needs kids.

You can find special needs kids playgroups through different autism groups, sometimes they will place flyers in OT or speech therapy offices. Ask around and if you can't find a group to join, arrange a playdate with another Autism Mom. It is the perfect opportunity for the kids to come together and the moms to have some time to chat.

Another idea is to go to a Sensory Friendly Film. AMC Theatre partnered with the Autism Society to offer sensory friendly movie showings. AMC's website states "We turn the lights up, and turn the sound down, so you can get up, dance, walk, shout or sing!" How cool is that?

Other forward thinking businesses that have a heart for individuals with special needs have similar events. Sky High Sports in Santa Clara, CA, has a special needs jump time every Tuesday. According to their website, Sky High Sports "turns off the music, dims the lights and dials down the distractions for the comfort of our guests."

For a long time, we didn't go out with non-special needs families because I didn't want to impose on them. My son's behavior is unpredictable: he seems fine at the moment, and then he may start yelling and jumping up and down. If we did go, either my husband or I would leave early with my son and the other would stay with our girls. I worried that my son's behavior may upset someone if he got too loud or if he spilled something (he likes to dump things out).

Then one day my friend told me to relax and not worry about it. It was her backyard, and she reassured me she wasn't worried about him getting loud. So, she encouraged us to all stay and hang out. It was then that I realized how important it is to maintain your true friendships. We all get busy with our lives, and sometimes, it seems easier to just do your own thing rather than meeting up with friends because of what your child may or may not do.

Over the years I have found that maintaining these special friendships has become meaningful in so many ways to my family and me. There are people in our lives who we truly enjoy spending time with, and they accept our son and his behaviors without judgment. In fact, I have learned a thing or two by watching how our friends' college and high school age kids interact with my son.

Anytime we hang out with these friends, my son gravitates towards their kids. At the beach, he will go with them to play in the water or leave the beach and hang out in the hotel Jacuzzi with them. They are seemingly un-phased if he gets loud or splashes a bit. I, on the other hand, try not to care what other people think, but I admit it still hurts when people give us strange looks. Seeing these young men hanging out with my son not only warms my heart, it reminds me that unconditional love and acceptance of my son is paramount to his happiness. And really isn't that what we all want?

With so much focus on the needs of the child, your free time can get derailed, and you can forget to make time for your spouse. This journey you're on with a child with special needs is filled with challenges you never thought of when you imagined yourself as a parent. Yet, here you are. And as crazy as things may seem at times, if you have a spouse or partner that you can share this journey with, do what you can to foster that relationship.

Here are some ideas for things that you can do with your significant other:

- Standing date nights—It can be once a week or once a month but it should be a night without your child.

- Movie or Netflix night—If getting a babysitter is difficult or too costly, set a date at home for when your child is asleep. I know this can be difficult with the lure of your computer or your to do list. But you will feel much more connected with your partner if you share a laugh together (or a cry depending on the movie you pick).

- Hangout time—Depending on the demands in your life, it can be hard to find 10 minutes to just sit and connect with each other. However, it is important for your relationship. If you have a balcony or porch that you can just sit and talk for a few minutes, it makes it a little more special than just talking at the dinner table.

- Enjoy activities together—And if you really want to ensure that you are fostering your relationship, think back to what you used to love doing together before you had kids. Did you like to go hiking together? Or were concerts your thing? Maybe you enjoyed going to comedy shows together? Hanging out at bookstores? Go and do something fun together!

- Go to bed together—Aim to go to bed at the same time a few times each week. Sometimes when you and your spouse are so overwhelmed with everything that you have going on, you get disconnected from those you love most. When our son was first diagnosed, I spent so much time online late at night, so my husband would be asleep long before me. He would wake up before me so our limited time together during the week became even more minimal. It's important to be mindful of how much time we spend with our spouse and making a point to go to bed at the same time is a nice way to stay connected.

Getting out of the house, maintaining true friendships, and spending time with your spouse seem like such simple things, but when you have a child with autism, these sound like luxuries that you don't have time for. I implore you to prioritize this area; it may take some creativity on your part, but you can do this, you must do this, in order to nurture yourself and thrive as a family.

If you don't make a point to spend time with these other people in your life, you risk losing a part of yourself. Yes you are a Mom, and it is of utmost importance for you to nurture your child. However, you need to nurture yourself as well, and when you spend time with people that you love, you will nurture your heart and have more to share with your child.

You are striving each day to help your child in every way that you know how and that's wonderful. Your child is lucky to have you as his Mom, someone who loves him no matter what and is willing to do whatever it takes to reach his full potential—whatever that potential may be. Take a moment to remember who you are. In addition to being his Mom, you are also a wife, a friend, a sister, a daughter, etc. As compelling as it feels to devote your entire existence to helping your child, other people in your life need you too, and you need them.

Even with the best of intentions, an all-consuming focus on your child will isolate you from those whom you love. They want to help and support you. If you cut yourself off from spending time with them, you will lose a part of yourself. You need that connection with your friends and your spouse to fill your heart as you are pouring so much of your heart into your child. So get out there and do something fun, spend time with your friends and your spouse, and remember how amazing you are.

Chapter 22
Final Thoughts and
My Wish for You

"Promise me you'll always remember:
You're braver than you believe,
and stronger than you seem,
and smarter than you think."
—Christopher Robin to Pooh, A.A. Milne

You have been busy learning from the experts how to best advocate for your child. You have organized your autism paperwork so that you know where everything is and you don't have to hunt for it. You now have a system for managing your email, the paper that comes into your life, and a place to get things out of your head so they're not wearing you down.

You also have routines in place to make your life a lot easier as it takes the guesswork out of what you need to do next. You have a plan for training your child on life skills and chores and have started streamlining your shopping so you have fewer errands to run.

Please be kind to yourself and don't berate yourself if you go off course at times. Certain things will resonate more with you than others, and it will seem effortless to implement those steps. Other steps that you try may be a little harder, even when you know that it is helping you. For me, I still have my alarm set to tell me to go to bed each night. It's been difficult breaking the habit of going to bed late even though I now love the feeling I get when I wake early in the morning before my family is up.

Gradually, I shifted my bed time a few minutes earlier each week. I now go to bed an hour earlier than my old bedtime, but I can still feel the temptation to stay up later. It is becoming less tempting as time goes by.

Breaking habits that don't serve your life's purpose and finding new ones is a vital component of being able to thrive.

Having a child with autism has taught me so many lessons and has reshaped my views on so many things. I have a deeper appreciation for the simple things in life, and as a family, we celebrate the smallest milestones because we know how hard we worked to reach them. Most of all, I have learned a lot about myself: I learned that I would do anything for my children even if it means going outside of my comfort zone.

As Autism Moms, our lives shouldn't be about managing chaos, although I know it feels that way sometimes. We are all members of the same club even though none of us signed up to join.

At the beginning of this book, I said the H.E.A.R.T. Method was designed to help Moms as we are the heart of our families and homes. As you implement the different steps, I hope you feel empowered to make positive changes in your life and feel buoyed by each small success. I hope you see how valuable you are as a Mom, and that despite the many challenges this diagnosis brings, your child is a gift to be treasured, and that's why you are working so hard to advocate for him.

The diagnosis is devastating at first, and it takes time for the pain of this to ease, but know that it doesn't mean that your child or your family will have a terrible life. You will put one step in front of the other; and, however, small your steps are, you will move forward, you will build a life for your child and your family to thrive.

As a parent of a child with autism, I feel your pain: the pain that comes from feeling like the plans and dreams you had for your child are slipping away, the world is falling apart around you without knowing what to do or where to turn, and wanting help but not knowing where to start. This book is your place to start. This is your guide to getting your child the help that he needs and also the help that you need to get your home, life and heart back in balance.

Today I hope that you will prioritize your self-care. Ultimately, if you don't take care of yourself, you will have little to give. You are an Autism Mom and you are the *heart* of your family. Be sure to get some rest, make small changes each day, enjoy your child each step of the way, and you will build a beautiful life.

Acknowledgments

When my son was diagnosed, I was overwhelmed and didn't know whom to talk to. My heartfelt thanks go out to Parents Helping Parents (a non-profit organization in San Jose) and Mary Burkhart. Mary facilitated the autism support group for Parents Helping Parents, and she was the first autism mom that I met. She helped me when I was feeling hopeless and told me one day I would do the same for other autism moms.

Over time I have met incredible women that have inspired me to write this book and help other autism moms. Gina Lukas, thank you for coming into my life at the perfect time and helping me when I was struggling. Meg Zucker, thank you for making this world a better place, your energy and enthusiasm inspire me. Thank you, Cassie Boorn, for being an inspirational coach that helped me find my purpose and helped me launch my blog when I didn't think I was ready. Thank you Lindsay Humes for helping me with the technical aspects of managing my blog, you really do know everything. Rachel Dool, thank you for all of your help and creativity, I would be lost without you.

I am so grateful for Eloisa Arenas for being there through all life's ups and downs, my life wouldn't be the same without you. Liz Longacre, thank you for adding so much insight during the writing process, we were destined to be friends. Thank you to my fellow Autism Moms—Lisa Valerio, La Donna Ford, Jean Lee and many others. Your support and input while I was writing this book was invaluable.

Many thanks to my editor, Katie Chambers, for your incredible editorial guidance. I felt very lucky to work with Jen Henderson of Wild Words Formatting, her immeasurable support and wisdom encouraged me in the final phases of this book.

Our family has been blessed with amazing teachers, administrators, and therapists that have touched our lives through the years. You have celebrated each high with us and supported us through every low. I thank you with all my heart for dedicating your life's work to helping children with autism and their families. You truly make a difference.

My family is grateful to have grandparents on both sides of our family as well as aunts and uncles that have supported us through this journey. Their unconditional love and support has given us strength when we needed it the most.

Thank you to my husband and children for understanding why I needed to write this book and supporting me through my writing journey. You have given me a greater life than I could ever have imagined.

Notes

Duhigg, Charles. The Power of Habit: Why We Do What We Do in Life and Business. New York: Random House, 2012.

Emmons, Richard A. How Gratitude Can Help You Through Hard Times. Greater Good: The Science of a Meaningful Life (Website). University of California Berkeley.

Fulton, Alice and Pauline Hatch. It's Here… Somewhere. Cincinnati, OH: Writer's Digest Books, 1991.

Kondo, Marie. The Life-Changing Magic of Tidying Up: The Japanese Art of Decluttering and Organizing. Ten Speed Press 2014.

McKeown, Greg. Essentialism: The Disciplined Pursuit of Less. New York: Crown Publishing, 2014.

Peale, Norman Vincent. The Power of Positive Thinking. Prentice-Hall. 1952.

Rubin, Gretchen. The Happiness Project: The Happiness Project: Or Why I Spent a Year Trying to Sing in the Morning, Clean My Closets, Fight Right, Read Aristotle, and Generally Have More Fun. New York: Harper, 2009.

Resources

Here are a few resources, please check my website (www.AutismMomMindset.com) as I will continually add resources there.

The Autism Society of America (www.autism-society.org). They have affiliates (chapters) across the country. Their website will help you locate the affiliate closest to you.

Center for Parent Information and Resources (www.parentcenterhub.org/find-your-center) – Find the Parent Training and Information (PTI) Center or Community Parent Resource Center (CPRC) near you. These organizations offer valuable information and support to parents of children with disabilities.

Community Gatepath (www.gatepath.org) located in Redwood City, California.

Don't Hide It Flaunt It (www.DontHideItFlauntIt.com) – a not-for-profit organization that works to advance understanding, tolerance and mutual respect for people's differences.

Environmental Working Group's Cosmetic Database (www.CosmeticsDatabase.com).

Healthy Kids Happy Kids (www.HealthyKidsHappyKids.com) – Online resource for trusted kids' health advice, fun tips, random thoughts and adventures with Dr. Elisa Song, holistic pediatrician and mama of two crazy fun kids.

Mental Health & Autism Insurance Project (www.autismhealthinsurance.org) – a non-profit public benefit corporation helps families secure health insurance and other coverage for mental health and autism related interventions.

Parents Helping Parents (www.php.com) located in San Jose, California. They offer emotional support and guidance, parent education and training, assistive technology preview and demonstration center, special needs library and more.

About the Author

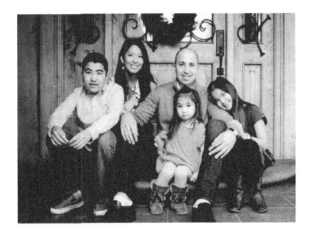

Katherine Kanaaneh utilizes the knowledge she gained through participating in and now facilitating an autism support group to help other parents navigate the world of autism—a world she has been learning to navigate for ten years. She vividly remembers the feelings of isolation, grief, and overwhelm when her son was first diagnosed with autism 10 years ago, and she feels lucky to have found a support group early on in her journey. With this support, she began to feel empowered; however, despite the empowerment, she still felt overwhelmed with everything on her plate. Thus, as a former CPA, she used her organizational skills and financial knowledge to help her cope with the paperwork overload. While she still plans to craft a children's book—the book she always thought she would write—using notes she jots down whenever one of her three children tells her stories, her primary focus is helping other autism moms as she manages her blog Autism Mom Mindset. By implementing the advice given in her Autism with HEART method, she was able to find time to enjoy activities she loves: spending time with family and friends, writing, reading, wine tasting, and keeping fit. She hopes you will set your intention to make one positive change daily: choose one tip found in the book each day to help regain control of your life. And always remember to go shine.

Connect with Katherine at the following places:

Website: www.AutismMomMindset.com
Facebook: www.facebook.com/AutismMomMindset
Twitter: www.twitter.com/Autism_Mindset

Thank you so much for reading this book. Would you kindly leave a review? Please take 2–3 minutes to leave a review on Amazon.

I truly appreciate it and wish you and your family all the best.

Go shine!

Kat =)

Made in the USA
Las Vegas, NV
18 September 2023

77768298R00111